HARMONIZE AND THRIVE

HARMONIZE AND THRIVE

A HOLISTIC GUIDE TO SYNCHRONIZING YOUR CYCLE AND WOMEN'S HORMONE HEALTH (2-IN-1 COLLECTION)

WOMEN'S HEALTH

LILA LACY

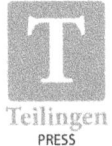

Teilingen
PRESS

Copyright © 2024 by Lila Lacy

All rights reserved. No part of this book may be reproduced, stored in a retrieval system, or transmitted in any form or by any means, electronic, mechanical, photocopying, recording, or otherwise, without the prior written permission of the publisher, Teilingen Press.

The information contained in this book is based on the author's personal experiences and research. While every effort has been made to ensure the accuracy of the information presented, the author and publisher cannot be held responsible for any errors or omissions.

This book is intended for general informational purposes only and is not a substitute for professional medical, legal, or financial advice. If you have specific questions about any medical, legal, or financial matters matters, you should consult with a qualified healthcare professional, attorney, or financial advisor.

Teilingen Press is not affiliated with any product or vendor mentioned in this book. The views expressed in this book are those of the author and do not necessarily reflect the views of Teilingen Press.

For every woman who has ever felt out of step with her own body, this book is for you. It's a guiding light for those days when you need a little extra help, a reminder that your body's rhythms are a dance you can learn.

May the pages within guide you to a deeper understanding of your body's wisdom, and empower you to find harmony within.

In the rhythm of the body, we find the melody of the mind and the harmony of the soul.

— ANONYMOUS

CONTENTS

Introduction   xi

SYNC YOUR CYCLE

Embracing the Power of Your Cycle   3
1. Understanding Your Menstrual Cycle   9
2. Nutrition and Your Cycle   19
3. Exercise and Your Cycle   29
4. Cycle Alignment in Your Personal Life   39
5. Cycle Alignment in Your Professional Life   47
6. Cycle Alignment and Fertility   53
7. Cycle Alignment for Health Conditions   63
8. Holistic Approaches to Cycle Alignment   71
9. Creating Your Personal Cycle Alignment Plan   81
10. The Future of Cycle Alignment   91

Your Journey Beyond the Pages   101

WOMAN'S HORMONE HANDBOOK

Embracing Hormonal Harmony   109
1. Understanding Hormones: The Basics   113
2. Puberty to Fertility: The Reproductive Years   123
3. Pregnancy and Hormones: The Miracle of Life   133
4. Perimenopause and Menopause: Transitioning Phases   143
5. Thyroid Health: The Metabolic Regulator   153
6. Stress and Hormones: The Adrenal Connection   163
7. Weight, Metabolism, and Hormones   173
8. Mood, Brain Function, and Hormones   183
9. Skin, Hair, and Hormones   193
10. Integrative Approaches to Hormone Health   203

Your Hormonal Journey   213

Epilogue   219

Your Feedback Matters 223
About the Author 225

INTRODUCTION

Welcome to "Harmonize and Thrive," a 2-in-1 collection crafted to guide you through the labyrinth of your own physiology, where the whispers of hormones become the language of self-awareness and empowerment. This book is a tribute to the everyday woman—the dreamer, the doer, the nurturer, and the warrior—offering a compass to navigate the intricate world of hormones, those unsung heroes orchestrating the vast symphony of womanhood.

These potent chemical messengers are pivotal in every chapter of a woman's life, from the awakening of puberty to the transformative waves of menopause. Every day and night, your hormones work harmoniously to create the rich and dynamic experience of being a woman. Hormones like estrogen and progesterone ebb and flow, shaping reproductive health and influencing everything from mood to metabolism.

"Sync Your Cycle," the first book in the collection, invites you to delve into the transformative power of cycle synchronization. Imagine a world where you can anticipate and harness the ebb and flow of your energy, aligning your daily habits with the phases of your menstrual cycle for optimal well-being. This guide offers a fresh perspective on embracing your body's cyclical wisdom, turning what society has often deemed a weakness into your greatest strength.

Introduction

The second book, "Woman's Hormone Handbook," is designed to illuminate the complex interactions of hormones with your body. In this book, we'll embark on an enlightening journey to decode the whispers and roars of your hormonal landscape, providing you with the knowledge to understand your body's signals and act upon them. Understanding these signals is crucial, as they influence not just physical health but also emotional well-being and mental clarity. As we unfold the pages of this guide, you'll gain insights into how to harmonize your body's natural rhythms, empowering you to live with vitality and grace.

Together, these books form a comprehensive manual for the modern woman. They are a testament to the resilience and adaptability of the female body and a celebration of the potential within each of us. "Harmonize and Thrive" is more than just a title—it's a philosophy, a way of life that acknowledges the profound connection between our physical cycles and overall quality of life.

As you journey through these pages, you will learn to navigate hormonal shifts with confidence, build a nourishing diet that supports each phase of your cycle, and adapt your fitness routine to work with your body's natural rhythms. You will discover how to foster deeper connections in your personal relationships through cycle awareness and elevate your productivity and energy levels at work by channeling peak energy and focus when it counts.

This collection is your personal roadmap to a more energized and balanced life. It is a call to action for any woman ready to harness her hormonal power and transform her life. Whether you are seeking to enhance your fertility, conquer menstrual woes, or simply live in greater harmony with your body, "Harmonize and Thrive" is the ultimate companion on your journey to self-discovery and well-being.

So, dear reader, prepare to embark on a transformative journey with "Harmonize and Thrive." Let this collection guide you to a life where every period is not a hindrance but a stepping stone to becoming the most vibrant version of yourself. Welcome to the dance of your biology, where every step is choreographed by the innate intelligence of your body.

SYNC YOUR CYCLE

HARNESS YOUR MENSTRUAL CYCLE FOR HORMONAL HARMONY AND HOLISTIC WELLNESS

EMBRACING THE POWER OF YOUR CYCLE

Imagine if you could tap into a hidden superpower—one that ebbs and flows just like the tides, governed by the moon's pull. Your menstrual cycle holds this power, a rhythmic dance of hormones that, when understood and honored, can elevate your well-being to new heights. This isn't just about managing your period; it's about embracing the full spectrum of your cycle's phases, each with its own secret code to unlock your body's potential.

Think of your cycle as a symphony, with each movement expressing a different mood and energy. By tuning into this natural rhythm, you can live your life with more grace and vitality. It's about aligning your daily habits—from the food you savor to the movements you enjoy—with the natural flow of your body's menstrual cycle. There are numerous names for this process of alignment, including cycle syncing, cycle awareness, cycle optimization and hormone-based living.

Embracing the Power of Your Cycle

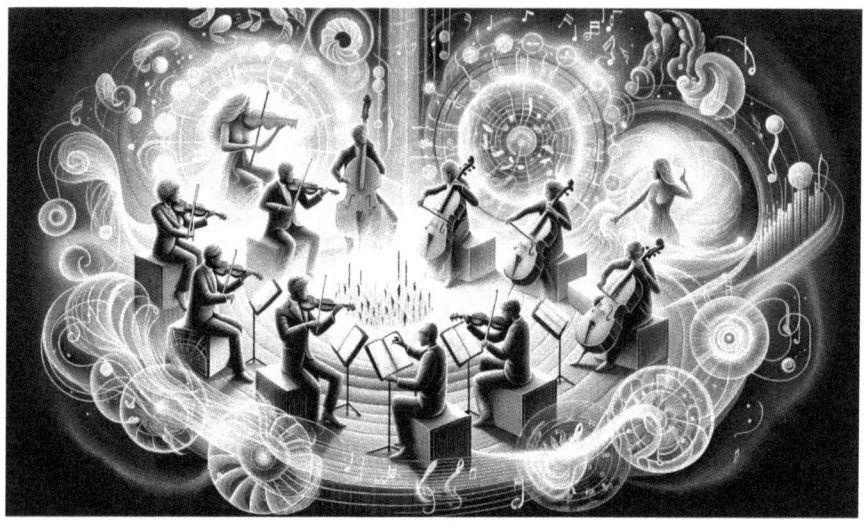

This journey into synchronizing your cycle is a path to empowerment. It's a call to listen intently to the whispers of your body and respond with nurturing care. As you learn to ride the waves of your hormonal shifts, you'll discover a profound connection with yourself that's both grounding and liberating.

The rewards of this alignment are as rich and varied as life itself. Women who embrace this wisdom often speak of a newfound zest for life, smoother cycles, and a clearer mind. It's a lifestyle that honors your body's innate wisdom, allowing you to move with the rhythms of nature rather than against them.

As we embark on this adventure together, we'll uncover the secrets of your cycle, transforming what you may have thought of as a monthly inconvenience into a source of strength and synchronization. You'll learn to make choices that resonate deeply with your body's needs, empowering you to live a life that's not just in sync with your cycle but also in tune with your truest self.

So, let's turn the page and begin this transformative journey. Your body is ready to reveal its secrets—are you ready to listen?

Self-Awareness and Body Wisdom

Step into the world of self-discovery, where the simple act of understanding your body becomes a radical act of self-care. In today's fast-paced society, we often become disconnected from the natural rhythms that govern our well-being. But imagine if you could reclaim that connection, tuning into the ebb and flow of your own biology with the finesse of a masterful conductor.

Your menstrual cycle is not just a biological process; it's a gateway to a deeper understanding of who you are. It's a monthly voyage that invites you to explore your body's inner workings, listen to its subtle cues, and respond with compassion and intelligence. This is where the magic happens—you begin to move in harmony with your intrinsic rhythms, and life unfolds more easily and synchronicity.

In embracing this dance of self-awareness, you're not just synchronizing your cycle; you're charting a course to a more empowered you. It's a journey that challenges the status quo and can help you live a life where your health and happiness are not left to chance but are consciously crafted with each phase of your cycle in mind.

This is about more than just surviving your menstrual cycle; it's about thriving within it. By becoming attuned to your body's signals, you unlock a wealth of knowledge that empowers you to make choices that support your physical, emotional, and mental health. It's an invitation to honor your body's natural wisdom, embrace its fluctuations, and celebrate its strength.

As we delve deeper into the art of aligning with your cycle, you'll find that this isn't just a practice; it's a reawakening. It's a call to reconnect with the most primal parts of yourself and to live a life that's not just balanced but vibrantly alive. So, take a deep breath and prepare to embark on a journey that will transform how you view your cycle, body, and potential.

Charting the Course of This Book

As we begin this journey together, let's unfold the map that will guide us through the rich terrain of your cycle. We'll navigate through the valleys and peaks of your hormonal landscape, discovering treasures of wisdom at every turn.

First, we'll embark on an expedition to understand the phases of your menstrual cycle, demystifying the science and the soul of your monthly rhythm. You'll learn to recognize the landmarks of your hormonal journey and how to harness their power.

Then, we'll explore nutrition and its impact on your cycle, where the foods you eat can become allies and nourish you in sync with the shifting tides of your hormones. We'll cultivate a feast that satisfies your palate and supports your cycle's unique nutritional needs. Exercise becomes an expression of self-love, a way to celebrate and strengthen your body in alignment with your cycle's phases. We'll provide guidance that can help you find the rhythm of movement that resonates with the beat of your body.

We'll then weave the wisdom of your cycle into the tapestry of your personal and professional life. You'll learn how to schedule and go about your days with the colors of your inner cycle, creating a masterpiece of balance and productivity.

We'll also touch on fertility, the healing potential for health conditions, and holistic cycle alignment approaches.

Armed with this new knowledge, you'll become the master of your own cycle and develop the confidence to create your cycle alignment habits that align with your life's unique contours. And finally, we'll gaze into the horizon at the future of cycle alignment, envisioning a world where every woman's cycle is a source of strength and empowerment.

This book is your invitation to a grand adventure, a call to journey inward and emerge with a profound connection to the ebb and flow of your own body. So lace up your boots, dear explorer—the path to syncing with your cycle awaits, and the possibilities are as boundless as your own potential.

Your Personal Odyssey: Navigating the Pages Ahead

As you stand at the start of this grand adventure, know that you are about to embark on a personal journey that promises to be as unique as you are. This book is not a one-size-fits-all manual but a treasure map to chart your course through the waters of cycle alignment.

Approach each chapter with curiosity and an open heart. You may choose to read this book from cover to cover, immersing yourself in the whole experience, or you may wish to navigate directly to the chapters that call out to you and resonate with the questions that bubble up from within you.

This is your adventure, and you are the captain. This book is a living document meant to be filled with your thoughts, reflections, and revelations. It is a space for you to converse with yourself, ask questions, and discover answers that are true to your soul.

And as you chart your journey, remember that this book is but one star in a constellation of resources. There may be companion guides, online communities, and workshops that serve as fellow travelers, offering support and camaraderie as you explore the wonders of your cycle.

So, take a deep breath, and prepare to embark on a journey of self-discovery that will transform not just how you view your cycle but how you live each day.

The future is a canvas stretched before you, and you hold the brush. Let the rhythm of your cycle be the stroke that guides you, painting a life that is as dynamic, beautiful, and profound as the journey you're about to undertake.

1
UNDERSTANDING YOUR MENSTRUAL CYCLE

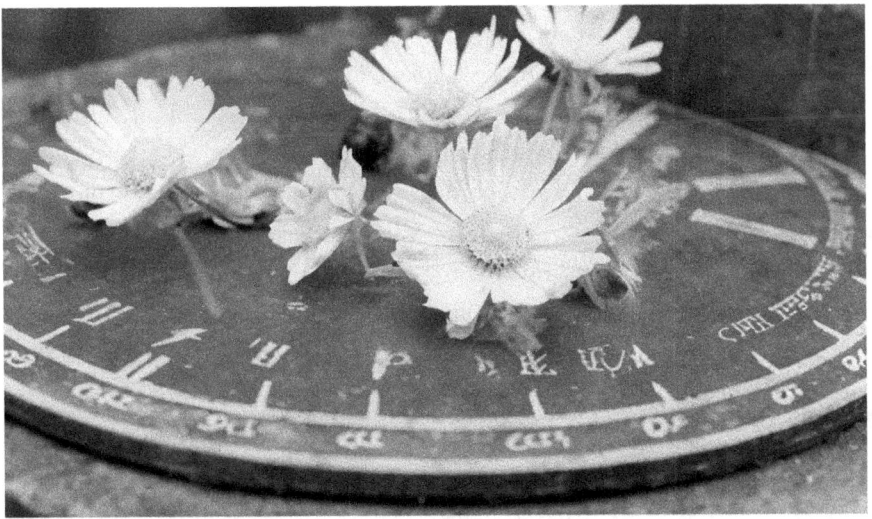

Embarking on the journey to understand your menstrual cycle is akin to unlocking a deeper level of self-awareness. The menstrual cycle is not just a biological process but a complex interplay of hormones that influence your physical health, emotional well-being, and overall lifestyle. To fully harness the power of your hormones and harmonize your daily habits with your cycle, it is essential first to understand the distinct phases of the menstrual cycle and the physiological changes they involve.

The menstrual cycle can be divided into four primary phases: the menstrual phase, the follicular phase, ovulation, and the luteal phase. Each phase is characterized by hormonal fluctuations and bodily responses that affect energy levels, mood, appetite, and overall well-being.

The menstrual phase marks the beginning of the cycle, where the lining of the uterus is shed if fertilization has not occurred. This phase is commonly known as your period and can last anywhere from a few days to a week. During this time, hormone levels, particularly estrogen and progesterone, are at their lowest, which can lead to the common symptoms of menstruation, such as cramps, fatigue, and mood swings. Many women report feeling more introspective and may benefit from gentle activities and nourishing foods during this time.

The follicular phase follows, and it typically culminates with the body preparing for ovulation. This phase can last about 7 to 10 days and is characterized by a rise in estrogen and follicle-stimulating hormone (FSH), which stimulates the growth of follicles in the ovaries and causes the uterine lining to thicken again in preparation for a potential pregnancy. This phase is often associated with increased energy, mental clarity, and creativity. Leveraging this time for brainstorming, planning, and engaging in more vigorous physical activities can be advantageous.

Ovulation is the pinnacle of the menstrual cycle, a brief but critical phase that usually occurs mid-cycle, around day 14 in a 28-day cycle. The surge in estrogen from the follicular phase leads to a spike in luteinizing hormone (LH), which triggers the release of an egg from the ovary into the fallopian tube. Estrogen peaks just before ovulation, and many women experience heightened senses, energy, and libido. This is when you are most fertile, and the body is primed for conception. Ovulation is often accompanied by physical signs such as a slight rise in basal body temperature and changes in cervical mucus. This phase can be an optimal time for socializing, high-intensity workouts, and critical decision-making.

Following ovulation, the ruptured follicle transforms into the corpus luteum, which secretes progesterone. Progesterone works in concert with estrogen to maintain the endometrial lining, creating a supportive environment for an embryo. If fertilization does not occur, the corpus luteum degenerates, leading to a drop in progesterone and estrogen levels. This hormonal shift causes the endometrial lining to shed, resulting in menstruation, and the cycle begins anew. During the luteal phase, some women may experience premenstrual symptoms. It's a period that may call for self-care, reflection, and preparation for the cycle to restart.

Understanding these phases and their hormonal changes is empowering. It allows for a deeper comprehension of your body's natural rhythms. By recognizing the ebb and flow of your hormonal landscape, you can tailor your nutrition, exercise, social life, and work tasks to harmonize with your body's flow. This alignment fosters a sense of harmony within and empowers you to make informed decisions that can enhance your productivity, vitality, energy, and wellbeing.

Cycle synchronization is not a one-size-fits-all approach; it's a personalized journey that evolves with you. It is about aligning with the body's natural state at any given time. It gives you the confidence to make informed choices that honor your body's needs, leading to a more balanced and fulfilled life.

Hormones and Their Functions

At the heart of cycle syncing is the endocrine system, which plays a pivotal role in regulating menstrual cycles. The endocrine system is a network of glands that secrete hormones directly into the bloodstream. These are all controlled by the hypothalamus, the brain's hormone control center. Your hormones, in turn, act as messengers, influencing various bodily functions, including reproduction, metabolism, and mood.

To truly understand and benefit from cycle alignment, we will explore the key hormones involved in your menstrual cycle, the functions they serve, and how their levels change throughout your cycle in more depth.

Estrogen

Estrogen is pivotal in the development of secondary sexual characteristics and the thickening of the uterine lining (endometrium) during the follicular phase in preparation for potential pregnancy. It also regulates the menstrual cycle and affects various other bodily systems.

Estrogen levels rise steadily during the follicular phase, peaking just before ovulation. After ovulation, levels drop sharply and rise slightly during the luteal phase before falling again before menstruation.

Progesterone

Progesterone is essential for maintaining the endometrium, which is necessary for the implantation of a fertilized egg and sustaining early pregnancy. It also helps regulate the menstrual cycle and affects mood and libido.

Progesterone levels remain low during the follicular phase and begin to rise after ovulation, reaching their peak in the middle of the luteal phase. If pregnancy does not occur, progesterone levels fall, leading to the shedding of the uterine lining and the start of menstruation.

Follicle-Stimulating Hormone (FSH)

FSH is crucial for the growth and maturation of ovarian follicles containing the eggs. It also stimulates the production of estrogen by the ovaries.

FSH levels increase at the beginning of the cycle, during the follicular phase, to stimulate follicle development. They peak early in the cycle and then decline as estrogen levels rise.

Luteinizing Hormone (LH)

LH triggers ovulation—the release of a mature egg from the ovary. It also stimulates progesterone production by the corpus luteum, the follicle remnant after the egg is released.

LH levels surge mid-cycle, leading to ovulation. This LH surge is brief but crucial for the release of the egg and the subsequent rise in progesterone during the luteal phase.

Testosterone

Although often considered a male hormone, testosterone is also present in females and plays a role in libido, bone health, and the maintenance of muscle mass. It can also influence mood and energy levels.

Testosterone levels are relatively constant but experience a slight increase around the time of ovulation, which can contribute to a rise in sexual desire during this phase of the cycle.

The interplay of all of these hormones is not only fundamental to reproductive health but also affects physical and emotional well-being. By tuning into these hormones and their fluctuations throughout your cycle, you can cultivate a sense of harmony and well-being that resonates with your body's intrinsic patterns. This knowledge empowers you to make informed decisions about your health and well-being, attuned to your body's natural rhythms. With this knowledge as a foundation, the next step is to explore the practical aspects of tracking the menstrual cycle, which will empower you to apply this understanding to your own life.

Tracking Your Cycle: Methods and Tools

The next step after learning about hormonal changes and their functions is tracking your cycle. This process is not only fundamental to the process of cycle synchronization but also vital for gaining insights into your health and well-being.

To start tracking your cycle, you'll need to become familiar with the different phases and the length of your menstrual cycle, which can vary from the typical 28-day cycle. The first day of bleeding is considered day one of your cycle, and tracking continues to the day before your next period begins. Here are some ways you can track your cycle:

- **Calendar:** One of the simplest methods to track your cycle is using a calendar. You can mark the first day of your period and count the days until your next period begins. This will give you the length of your cycle. Additionally, you can note any symptoms you experience, such as cramps, mood swings, or changes in energy levels, which can indicate hormonal fluctuations.
- **Cycle tracking applications:** If you prefer to use technology, there are numerous apps available that can assist with cycle tracking. These apps often provide additional features such as reminders, symptom tracking, and predictions for fertile windows, which can be particularly useful for those trying to conceive or avoid pregnancy.
- **Basal body temperature:** Another tool for tracking your cycle is basal body temperature (BBT) charting. Your BBT is your body's temperature at rest and can be an indicator of ovulation. After ovulation, progesterone causes a slight increase in BBT. By tracking this temperature daily, you can see patterns and identify the ovulatory phase of your cycle.
- **Cervical mucus observation:** The consistency and amount of cervical mucus changes throughout your cycle due to hormonal variations. By tracking these changes, you can learn to recognize the fertile phase of your cycle.
- **Hormone tests:** Hormone testing kits are available for those seeking a more in-depth analysis. These kits can measure hormone levels in your urine to provide information about your cycle, such as when you enter your fertile window or confirm if ovulation has occurred.

It's important to note that while these methods can be very effective, they require consistency and attention to detail. Becoming comfortable with tracking and noticing patterns may take a few cycles. However, the insights gained from this practice can be incredibly empowering. By understanding your body's natural rhythms, you can make more informed decisions about your health, plan your schedule to align with your cycle phases and optimize your well-being.

As you become more attuned to your body's signals and the nuances of your menstrual cycle, you'll be better prepared to delve into the science of cycle alignment and harmonize your lifestyle with the ebbs and flows of your hormonal landscape. This knowledge is a foundation for the next steps in your journey toward a more synchronized and harmonious existence with your body.

Common Myths and Misconceptions

In the journey to understand and harness the power of our menstrual cycles, it is crucial to dismantle the barriers of misinformation that often cloud our perception of them. These can range from benign misunderstandings to deeply ingrained stereotypes.

One common myth is that the menstrual cycle only affects a person's mood. While it is true that hormonal fluctuations can influence emotions, the impact of the menstrual cycle is far more comprehensive, affecting physical energy, cognitive function, and even nutritional needs. To view the cycle through the narrow lens of mood swings alone is to overlook the intricate symphony of changes within the body.

Another misconception is that cycle optimization is solely about fertility and contraception. While understanding the menstrual cycle is undoubtedly beneficial for family planning, cycle syncing extends its benefits to various aspects of health and well-being, including stress management, exercise optimization, and dietary adjustments. It is a holistic approach that acknowledges the cyclical nature of the female body.

There is also the mistaken belief that all menstrual cycles are uniform and should conform to a 28-day standard. In reality, cycles can vary significantly in length and characteristics, with a healthy range typically falling between 21 and 35 days. The notion of a "perfect" cycle can lead to unnecessary anxiety and a misalignment between one's unique rhythm and the generalized cycle alignment recommendations.

Furthermore, some may believe that cycle optimization is an unscientific practice rooted more in new-age philosophy than empirical evidence. However, a growing body of research supports the physiological basis for the practice, highlighting the importance of tailoring lifestyle choices to the menstrual cycle's phases to enhance overall health and quality of life.

Lastly, there is the misconception that cycle synchronization is only for those who experience regular cycles. Even individuals with irregular cycles or conditions such as polycystic ovary syndrome (PCOS) can benefit from understanding their body's signals and patterns. Cycle syncing is not a one-size-fits-all solution but a personalized approach that can be adapted to each individual's unique circumstances.

We can pave the way for a more informed and empowered approach to cycle alignment by dispelling these myths and misconceptions. Through this clarity, individuals can truly harness the potential of their menstrual cycles, not only to optimize their daily lives but also to foster a deeper connection with their bodies.

Chapter Summary

- The menstrual cycle is a complex interplay of hormones affecting health and lifestyle, and understanding it can lead to greater self-awareness and well-being.
- The cycle consists of four phases: menstrual, follicular, ovulation, and luteal, each with distinct hormonal changes and bodily responses.
- The menstrual phase involves shedding the uterine lining, with low hormone levels causing symptoms like cramps and mood swings.
- The follicular phase sees rising estrogen levels as ovarian follicles mature, preparing the uterus for potential pregnancy.

- Ovulation is the release of an egg due to a hormone surge, marking the peak of fertility with physical signs like a rise in basal body temperature.
- The luteal phase involves the secretion of progesterone from the corpus luteum to maintain the uterine lining, with the cycle restarting if no fertilization occurs.
- Hormones like FSH, LH, estrogen, and progesterone guide the menstrual cycle, influencing fertility, mood, and overall health.
- Tracking the menstrual cycle using calendars, apps, BBT charting, cervical mucus observation, or hormone testing kits can empower individuals to align their lifestyles with their cycle phases.
- Cycle synchronization involves aligning diet, exercise, and activities with the menstrual cycle's phases for improved health and harmony.
- Common myths about the menstrual cycle include its impact being limited to mood, its relevance only for fertility, the existence of a "perfect" cycle length, and the dismissal of cycle syncing as unscientific.

2

NUTRITION AND YOUR CYCLE

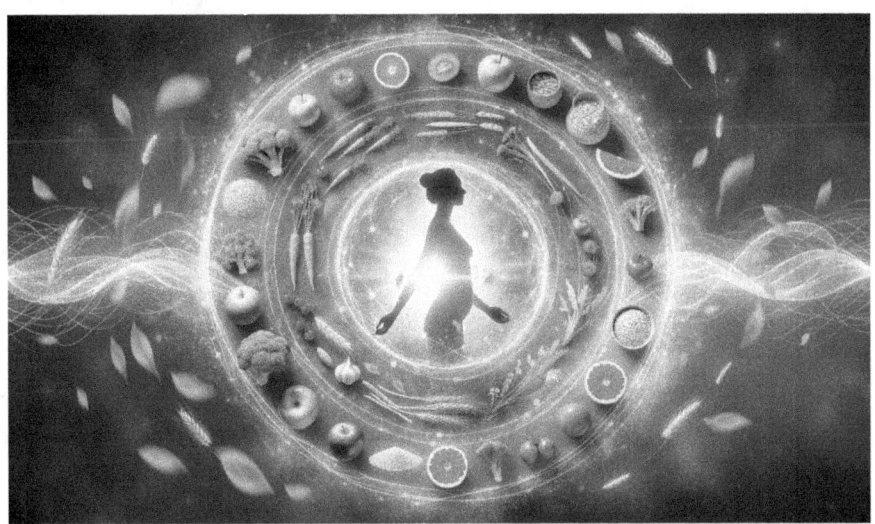

A s we begin to explore nutrition and how it relates to your menstrual cycle, it is essential to understand your body's changing nutritional demands during each phase.

Eating for Your Menstrual Phase

As we explored in the last chapter, the menstrual phase marks the beginning of your cycle and is characterized by the shedding of the uterine lining. It can be accompanied by symptoms such as cramps, fatigue, and mood swings and is a period that requires special attention to dietary choices to support your body's needs.

During the menstrual phase, your body is in a state of release and renewal. Iron levels can be particularly impacted due to blood loss, making it crucial to replenish this vital nutrient. Foods rich in iron, like leafy greens, legumes, red meat, poultry, and fish, should be incorporated into your meals. Pair these foods with those high in vitamin C, like citrus fruits, bell peppers, and berries, to enhance iron absorption. This synergistic effect maximizes iron uptake and supports your immune system.

In addition to iron, your body will benefit from foods high in omega-3 fatty acids. These essential fats, found in flaxseeds, walnuts, and fatty fish like salmon, can help manage inflammation and alleviate menstrual cramps. They also influence mood regulation, which can be particularly beneficial if you experience emotional shifts during this phase.

Complex carbohydrates are another critical component of eating for your menstrual phase. Whole grains, such as brown rice, quinoa, and oats, provide sustained energy and are rich in B vitamins, essential for energy production and the health of your nervous system. These complex carbs also contribute to a feeling of fullness and can help stabilize blood sugar levels, curbing cravings and mood swings.

Hydration is paramount during the menstrual phase. Drinking plenty of water helps to replace fluids lost during menstruation and can aid in reducing bloating. Herbal teas, such as ginger or peppermint, can offer additional comfort, easing digestive discomfort and soothing cramps.

Lastly, listening to your body's signals during this time is important. If you experience cravings, it's not uncommon to seek out comfort in the form of food. While it's perfectly acceptable to indulge mindfully, aim to maintain a balance by choosing nutrient-dense snacks like dark chocolate, which is high in magnesium. This mineral can relax muscles and ease cramping.

Focusing on these nutritional strategies during the menstrual phase supports your body's natural processes and sets a strong foundation for the remainder of your cycle. With thoughtful food choices, you can navigate this phase with greater ease and comfort, readying yourself for the transition into the next phase of your cycle, where different nutritional considerations will come into play.

Eating for Your Follicular Phase

As we transition from the menstrual phase into the follicular phase of your cycle, your body embarks on a new beginning. This phase, typically lasting from about day 7 to day 14 of your cycle, is characterized by the body's preparation for potential pregnancy. It's a time when the follicles in the ovaries mature and estrogen levels rise. With this physiological shift, your nutritional needs also evolve.

The follicular phase is an opportune moment to support your body with foods that enhance estrogen production and follicle growth. A diet rich in phytoestrogens can be particularly beneficial during this time. Phytoestrogens are plant-derived compounds that can mimic the effects of estrogen in the body, and they can be found in foods such as flaxseeds, soybeans, and legumes. Incorporating these into your meals can help balance your hormones naturally.

As estrogen levels increase, so does your body's capacity to build muscle. The follicular phase is excellent for focusing on foods rich in high-quality proteins. Think lean meats, fish, eggs, and plant-based sources like quinoa and lentils. These will support muscle growth and repair and provide sustained energy levels.

Your energy levels are likely to be higher during the follicular phase, and your metabolism may also start to speed up. Complex carbohydrates are your allies to match this increased energy demand. They provide a steady release of energy, perfect for keeping you fueled throughout the day. Foods such as sweet potatoes, oats, and whole grains are excellent choices.

Moreover, the follicular phase is when your body is more insulin-sensitive, meaning it's better at utilizing carbohydrates for energy rather than storing them as fat. This makes it a strategic time to include moderate portions of healthy carbohydrates.

Antioxidants are also crucial during this phase to help protect the developing follicle from oxidative stress. Brightly colored fruits and vegetables, such as berries, citrus fruits, and leafy greens, are packed with vitamins and antioxidants. They not only support overall health but also contribute to the health of your reproductive system.

In addition to specific food groups, certain vitamins and minerals deserve special attention during the follicular phase. Vitamin E, found in nuts and seeds, can support the growth of the uterine lining. B vitamins, particularly B6 and B9, are essential for hormone balance and can be found in abundance in legumes, whole grains, and dark leafy vegetables.

Lastly, hydration remains a cornerstone of good health. Consuming ample water throughout the day will aid nutrient transport and overall cellular function.

By aligning your nutrition with your follicular phase, you are not only nurturing your body's immediate needs but also setting the stage for a healthier cycle overall. Remember, the key is to listen to your body and provide it with the nutrients required to thrive during each unique phase of your cycle.

Eating for Your Ovulatory Phase

As we transition from the follicular phase into the ovulatory phase of your menstrual cycle, your nutritional needs subtly shift in response to the hormonal changes within your body. The ovulatory phase, typically spanning 3 to 5 days, is characterized by a peak in luteinizing hormone (LH) and follicle-stimulating hormone (FSH), leading to the release of an egg from the ovary. This is a time of heightened fertility and energy, and your diet can play a supportive role in optimizing your well-being during this phase.

During ovulation, estrogen levels are at their highest, sometimes leading to a slight dip in appetite. However, it's essential to maintain a balanced diet to support your body's increased metabolic rate and the potential for conception if that is your goal.

To harness the full potential of your ovulatory phase through nutrition, focus on incorporating foods rich in fiber, antioxidants, and lean protein. These nutrients support the detoxification processes in the liver, which is vital for metabolizing and excreting excess estrogen.

Fiber-rich foods, such as leafy greens, berries, and legumes, are particularly beneficial during this time. They not only aid in digestion but also help regulate blood sugar levels, which can be particularly sensitive due to hormonal fluctuations. Aim for a variety of colorful vegetables and fruits, as they are packed with antioxidants that protect your cells from oxidative stress and support overall reproductive health.

Lean proteins, including fish, chicken, and plant-based options like lentils and chickpeas, provide the amino acids necessary for muscle repair and growth. These proteins are also vital for producing hormones and enzymes that play a role in the ovulatory process.

Additionally, foods rich in B vitamins, such as whole grains and dark leafy vegetables, can be particularly supportive. Vitamin B6, for instance, plays a role in synthesizing neurotransmitters, which can help maintain a positive mood and energy levels.

Omega-3 fatty acids in fatty fish like salmon, flaxseeds, and walnuts are also beneficial during ovulation. They contribute to the health of the cell membranes, which can be beneficial for egg quality and hormonal balance.

Hydration remains a crucial component of your diet during this phase. Adequate water intake is essential for maintaining the health of your cervical mucus, which is vital for fertility. Aim to drink plenty of water throughout the day, and consider incorporating hydrating foods like cucumbers, watermelon, and citrus fruits.

While the ovulatory phase is relatively short, it's a powerful time window in your cycle. You can support your overall health and vitality by choosing foods that align with your body's natural rhythms. Everyone's body is unique, and listening to your needs and responding is essential. If you have specific dietary restrictions or health concerns, consulting with a healthcare provider or a registered dietitian can provide personalized guidance to optimize your nutrition during this phase of your cycle.

As we explore the intricate relationship between your diet and your menstrual cycle, we will next delve into the nutritional strategies that can support you during the luteal phase, when your body prepares for either pregnancy or the onset of menstruation.

Eating for Your Luteal Phase

As we transition from the ovulatory phase of your menstrual cycle, we enter the luteal phase, which usually spans from day 15 to 28 of a typical 28-day cycle. This phase is characterized by the corpus luteum's release of progesterone, which prepares the body for a potential pregnancy. The luteal phase can often bring about various physical and emotional changes, including premenstrual symptoms. During this time, thoughtful nutrition can play a pivotal role in supporting your body's needs.

During the luteal phase, your metabolism may slightly increase, and you might experience heightened hunger. This is a natural response as your body's energy requirements grow. Increase your caloric intake slightly to accommodate this increased requirement, focusing on nutrient-dense foods that provide sustained energy and support hormonal balance.

Complex carbohydrates are particularly beneficial during this phase. Foods such as sweet potatoes, quinoa, brown rice, and oats can help maintain blood sugar levels and provide the necessary B vitamins that aid in the production of serotonin. This neurotransmitter promotes feelings of well-being and can be particularly helpful if you're experiencing mood swings.

Incorporating a variety of high-fiber foods is also crucial. Fiber helps regulate blood sugar and can aid in digestion, which can sometimes become sluggish during the luteal phase. Vegetables like brussels sprouts, broccoli, leafy greens, legumes, and seeds are excellent fiber sources.

Protein intake should remain consistent, focusing on lean proteins such as chicken, turkey, fish, tofu, and legumes. These proteins provide the amino acids necessary for neurotransmitter production, which can help mitigate some of the emotional changes that may occur during this time.

Healthy fats are another cornerstone of eating for your luteal phase. Foods rich in omega-3 fatty acids, such as salmon, flaxseeds, walnuts, and chia seeds, support cellular health and can help reduce inflammation, which may alleviate some premenstrual symptoms.

Magnesium-rich foods like dark chocolate, avocados, nuts, and seeds can be particularly beneficial. Magnesium plays a role in muscle relaxation and may help ease cramps and tension. It's also involved in synthesizing hormones and can support a sense of calm and relaxation.

Hydration remains essential throughout your cycle, but it's especially important to focus on during the luteal phase when some women experience bloating. Drinking plenty of water can reduce water retention and support overall bodily functions.

Lastly, listening to your body's cues during this phase is important. Craving certain foods during your luteal phase may indicate that your body is seeking specific nutrients. Honor these cravings within the context of a balanced diet, and remember that moderation is vital.

By aligning your nutritional choices with the needs of your luteal phase, you can support your body's natural rhythms and potentially ease some of the symptoms associated with this time of the month. In the following section, we will delve into how supplements can further complement cycle alignment efforts, offering additional support to your overall well-being throughout your menstrual cycle.

Supplements and Your Cycle

In aligning your nutrition with your menstrual cycle, understanding the role of supplements is a vital piece of the puzzle. While whole foods should always be the cornerstone of your diet, certain supplements can support your body's unique needs throughout the different phases of your cycle.

As we delve further into the concept of cycle alignment, it's essential to recognize that a delicate interplay of hormones governs each phase of your menstrual cycle. These hormones regulate your cycle and influence your energy levels, mood, and overall well-being. Supplements, when used thoughtfully and under a healthcare professional's guidance, can help optimize this hormonal balance and support your body's natural rhythms.

During the follicular phase, which begins after menstruation, your body is preparing for the possibility of pregnancy. Estrogen levels rise, leading to increased energy and a more robust metabolism. B-complex vitamins can be particularly beneficial to support this phase. They play a crucial role in energy production and can help maintain steady energy levels. Additionally, antioxidants like Vitamin E and selenium can support egg health, which is paramount during this time.

As you transition into the ovulatory phase, the body focuses on releasing an egg for potential fertilization. This is when you might feel at your most energetic and communicative. To support this phase, consider supplements that support hormonal balance and fertility, such as omega-3 fatty acids, which can aid in producing healthy cervical fluid.

Following ovulation, you enter the luteal phase, which we've previously discussed in the context of nutrition. During this time, progesterone becomes the dominant hormone. This shift can sometimes lead to premenstrual symptoms. Magnesium is a supplement that can be particularly helpful during the luteal phase. It plays a role in mood regulation, can alleviate cramps, and supports sleep. Additionally, Vitamin B6 can aid in synthesizing neurotransmitters like serotonin, which may help reduce mood swings and support overall emotional well-being.

Finally, during menstruation, your body is shedding the uterine lining and resetting for the next cycle. Iron is a crucial supplement during this phase, especially for those who experience heavy bleeding, as it helps to replenish the iron lost during menstruation. Vitamin C can aid in iron absorption, so pairing these two can be particularly effective.

It's crucial to remember that supplements are not a one-size-fits-all solution. The doses and combinations should be tailored to your health profile and the specific needs of each phase of your menstrual cycle. Always consult a healthcare provider before starting any new supplement regimen to ensure it's appropriate for your health status and goals.

By integrating supplements into your cycle-syncing practice, you can provide your body with the targeted support to thrive throughout each phase of your menstrual cycle. In conjunction with a balanced diet, this can empower you to harness the natural ebb and flow of your hormones, leading to improved health and vitality.

Chapter Summary

- The menstrual phase requires dietary choices that support the body's needs, including iron-rich foods and vitamin C to enhance iron absorption.
- Omega-3 fatty acids can help manage inflammation and mood swings, while complex carbohydrates provide sustained energy and stabilize blood sugar levels.
- Hydration is crucial, with water and herbal teas aiding in fluid replacement and reducing bloating, and listening to the body's signals for cravings is essential.
- The follicular phase benefits from foods that enhance estrogen production and muscle growth, including phytoestrogens, high-quality proteins, and complex carbohydrates.
- Antioxidants and specific vitamins like E and B support overall health and hormone balance during the follicular phase.
- The ovulatory phase requires a balanced diet with fiber, antioxidants, and lean protein to support metabolic rate and detoxification.
- The luteal phase may increase hunger and metabolism, requiring complex carbohydrates, high-fiber foods, lean proteins, and healthy fats to support the body.
- Supplements can complement cycle-syncing efforts, with specific vitamins and minerals supporting each menstrual cycle phase under healthcare guidance.

3

EXERCISE AND YOUR CYCLE

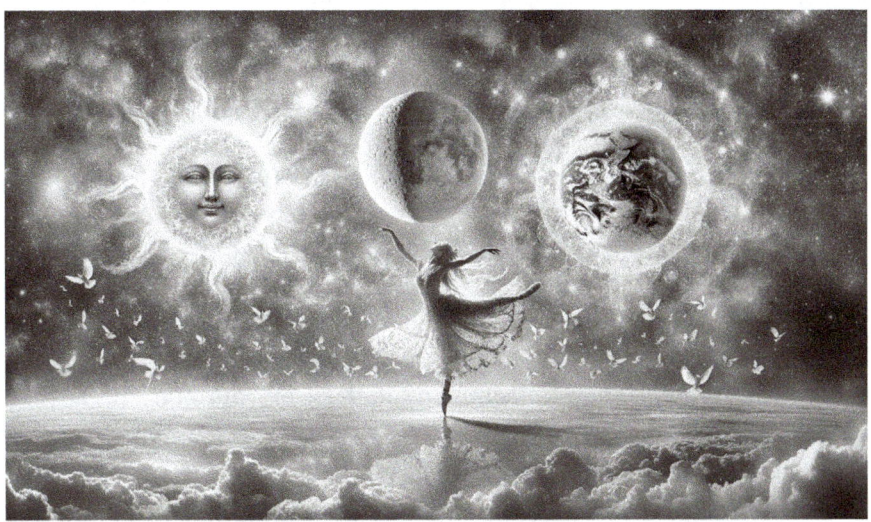

Recognizing the subtle yet informative cues your body provides throughout your menstrual cycle and adapting your workouts to these cues can maximize the benefits you reap from physical exercise. This attunement is the cornerstone of personalizing your fitness routine to harmonize with your cycle.

Adapting Workouts to Your Menstrual Phase

As we delve into the intricacies of cycle synchronization, particularly concerning exercise, it is essential to understand how the menstrual phase of your cycle can influence your workout regimen. During your menstrual phase, your body is shedding the uterine lining, accompanied by symptoms such as cramps, fatigue, and a general feeling of heaviness.

Given these physiological changes, it can help to adapt your exercise routine to accommodate your body's current state. This is not only a matter of comfort, but also one of harnessing the natural rhythm of your energy levels to optimize your fitness outcomes.

During the menstrual phase, your hormone levels—specifically estrogen and progesterone—are at their lowest. This hormonal state can lead to a decrease in energy and strength, making it an opportune time to engage in gentler, restorative workouts. Consider incorporating activities such as:

- **Yoga:** Gentle yoga flows can help to alleviate cramps and soothe your nervous system. Focus on comforting and restorative poses, such as child's pose, cat-cow stretches, and supine twists. These can help ease tension in the lower back and abdominal areas, often where discomfort is most pronounced during menstruation.
- **Walking:** A low-impact activity like walking can maintain your fitness without placing undue stress on your body. It's a form of exercise that can be easily adjusted to your energy levels—whether that means a leisurely stroll or a brisk walk.
- **Swimming:** If you're comfortable with it, swimming can be an excellent way to exercise during your period. The buoyancy of the water supports your body, and the gentle resistance can help maintain muscle tone without the strain of weight-bearing activities.
- **Pilates:** Pilates can help maintain core strength and stability with a low impact on your body. Focusing on breathing and

controlled movements is also beneficial for managing menstrual discomfort.

It's essential to listen to your body during this phase. Light resistance training or a shorter, less intense version of your regular workout might still be appropriate if you feel up to it. However, if your body is signaling the need for rest, honor that. Rest is a critical fitness component, and your body is already working hard during menstruation.

Hydration and proper nutrition are also vital during this phase. Ensure you're drinking plenty of water and eating nutrient-rich foods that can help replenish lost minerals and provide energy.

Remember, the goal of adapting your workouts to your menstrual phase is not to push through discomfort but to align your exercise routine with your body's natural feeling. By doing so, you can maintain your fitness while nurturing your body through the menstrual phase, setting a solid foundation for the more active phases of your cycle.

Adapting Workouts to Your Follicular Phase

As we transition from the menstrual phase into the follicular phase of your cycle, your energy levels begin to rise. This is a time when the body is primed for new beginnings and growth, both metaphorically and physiologically.

During this phase, estrogen levels start to climb, leading to increased energy, better mood, and often a heightened pain threshold. It's an ideal time to capitalize on these physiological changes by adapting your workout routine to match your body's changes. Your follicular is an ideal time to do activities like:

- **Strength training and muscle building:** The rising estrogen levels contribute to a boost in energy and aid in muscle repair and recovery. This makes the follicular phase an ideal time to focus on strength training. You may find that you can lift heavier weights or perform more repetitions than at other

times in your cycle. Incorporate exercises such as squats, deadlifts, and bench presses to build strength and muscle mass. Remember to start with challenging yet manageable weights and progressively increase the load to ensure continuous improvement.
- **Cardiovascular endurance:** Your body's increasing endurance capabilities during the follicular phase make it a great time to engage in more intense cardiovascular activities. Consider adding in running, cycling, or high-intensity interval training (HIIT) sessions. These workouts can help improve your cardiovascular health and take advantage of the natural upswing in your stamina.

As your body is generally less sensitive to pain and discomfort during this phase, it's also beneficial to continue working on flexibility and balance. Incorporate yoga or pilates into your routine to enhance your core strength, flexibility, and balance. These practices support your physical health and can contribute to mental clarity and stress reduction.

With the increase in energy and confidence, the follicular phase is a perfect time to set new fitness goals or try out activities you've been curious about. Whether it's a new fitness class, a challenging hike, or a dance workshop, your body is in an optimal state to embrace and adapt to new physical challenges.

Despite the inclination to push harder during this phase, listening to your body and incorporating adequate rest and recovery is crucial. Ensure you're allowing time for your muscles to repair by taking rest days as needed and engaging in active recovery activities such as light walking or stretching.

To support your increased activity levels, focus on a nutrient-rich diet that includes a balance of carbohydrates for energy, proteins for muscle repair, and healthy fats for hormone production.

By aligning your exercise regimen with the follicular phase of your cycle, you can harness the natural ebb and flow of your energy and hormonal levels. This synchronization optimizes your workouts for better performance and results and fosters a deeper connection with your body's innate wisdom.

Adapting Workouts to Your Ovulatory Phase

As we delve into the ovulatory phase of your menstrual cycle, it's essential to understand how this phase can influence your exercise regimen. The ovulatory phase is when your body is at its peak in terms of energy and physical performance due to a surge in hormones, particularly estrogen and luteinizing hormone. This hormonal shift can significantly impact your workout potential and recovery. You could consider workouts such as:

- **High-intensity and high-impact workouts:** During this phase, your body is primed for high-intensity and high-impact workouts. You may have more stamina, strength, and coordination, making it an excellent time to engage in activities that require power and endurance. This is the phase where you can push your limits and perhaps even set personal records.
- **Strength training:** Strength training during the ovulatory phase can be particularly effective. Due to the peak in estrogen, your muscles are more responsive, and you may experience increased muscle strength and peak power. It's a great time to focus on lifting heavier weights or performing more challenging resistance exercises. However, it's crucial to maintain proper form to prevent injury, as ligaments can be more lax due to hormonal fluctuations.
- **Cardiovascular exercise:** Cardiovascular exercises can also be intensified during this time. Consider incorporating sprint intervals, hill repeats, or high-intensity interval training (HIIT) sessions. These workouts can capitalize on your body's heightened energy levels and improved cardiovascular efficiency.

Group fitness classes or team sports can also be enjoyable and beneficial during ovulation. The social aspect of these activities aligns well with the increased communication skills and confidence often accompanying this phase of your cycle. Engaging with others in a workout setting can provide additional motivation and a sense of camaraderie.

While it's a time to take advantage of your body's peak performance, listening to your body's signals is also essential. Ensure you incorporate adequate warm-up routines to prepare your muscles and joints for intense activity, and don't neglect cool-down periods to aid recovery.

The ovulatory phase presents an opportunity to challenge yourself with higher-intensity workouts, capitalize on your body's increased strength and stamina, and enjoy the social aspects of exercise. By tuning into your body's rhythm and adapting your exercise routine to align with the ovulatory phase, you can optimize your fitness outcomes while honoring the natural rhythm of your cycle.

Adapting Workouts to Your Luteal Phase

As we delve into the luteal phase of your menstrual cycle, it's important to recognize that a shift in energy levels and physical sensations can characterize this period. The luteal phase involves significant hormonal changes that can influence your exercise routine and overall well-being.

During the luteal phase, progesterone levels rise, preparing the body for a potential pregnancy. This increase in progesterone and fluctuating estrogen levels can lead to feelings of bloating, fatigue, and sometimes a decrease in endurance. It's a time when your body is working hard internally, and as such, it may require a different approach to exercise compared to the more energetic ovulatory phase. To adapt your workouts to your luteal phase, consider incorporating the following:

- **Moderate-intensity activities:** These activities support your body's natural rhythms without overtaxing it. Strength training can be particularly beneficial during this time, as it helps maintain muscle mass and bone density. Focus on

moderate weights and higher repetitions rather than striving for personal bests or heavy lifting, which can be more challenging as your energy may not be at its peak.
- **Gentle movement:** Gentle movement practices such as yoga or pilates can be excellent choices. These forms of exercise emphasize core strength, flexibility, and relaxation, which can be soothing if you're experiencing premenstrual symptoms. The mindful breathing techniques used in these practices can also help manage any stress or mood swings that may arise due to hormonal fluctuations.

If your energy levels are still relatively high, consider continuing with cardiovascular exercises like brisk walking or light jogging. However, avoiding high-intensity interval training (HIIT) or prolonged strenuous activities that could exacerbate fatigue or stress the body unnecessarily during this phase can be helpful.

Above all, listening to your body and respecting its signals is essential. If you're feeling particularly tired or experiencing stronger premenstrual symptoms, it may be a sign to scale back the intensity or duration of your workouts. Restorative activities, such as leisurely walks or stretching sessions, can be just as valuable for your health and well-being during this time.

With its unique demands, the luteal phase offers an opportunity to practice self-care and mindfulness as you engage in physical activity. Remember, the goal is to support your body's needs, not push against them, ensuring you maintain a harmonious balance between movement and rest.

Listening to Your Body: Signs and Signals

The dialogue between your body's signals and your exercise choices is an ongoing process that requires patience, observation, and responsiveness.

Firstly, it is essential to recognize that your body's signs and signals are unique to you. They serve as a personal guide to optimizing your workouts. These signals can manifest in various forms, such as energy levels, muscle fatigue, mood fluctuations, and even sleep quality. By paying close attention to these indicators, you can tailor your exercise intensity and type to align with your body's needs at different phases of your cycle.

During the follicular phase, when estrogen levels rise, you might notice a surge in energy and strength. This is an opportune time to engage in more intense and challenging workouts, such as high-intensity interval training (HIIT) or strength training. Conversely, as you transition into the luteal phase, you may observe an energy shift, prompting you to consider more moderate or therapeutic activities, such as yoga or light cardio.

It is also vital to heed the signals of premenstrual syndrome (PMS), which can include bloating, headaches, and mood swings. These symptoms can affect your motivation and comfort during exercise. Adjusting your routine to include gentle movement and stretching can alleviate some of these discomforts and help maintain consistency in your fitness journey.

Moreover, during your menstrual phase, you might experience cramps and lower back pain, which are clear indicators that your body is asking for rest and recovery. This is a time to honor your body's request for gentler practices, perhaps focusing on activities like walking or Pilates, which can help maintain circulation without overexertion.

Listening to your body also means recognizing when you are capable of more than you might initially think. There may be days within each phase of your cycle when you feel powerful and resilient. Embrace these moments by challenging yourself while remaining within the boundaries of what feels right for your body.

In addition to physical signs, emotional and mental signals are equally important. Your mental state can significantly influence your physical performance and vice versa. Acknowledging and respecting your emotional well-being can guide you in choosing an exercise that benefits your body and uplifts your spirit.

Keeping a journal can be incredibly beneficial to facilitate this process of listening. Documenting your physical sensations, emotional state, and energy levels in relation to your cycle can help you discern patterns and make more informed decisions about your exercise regimen.

Remember that cycle alignment is not a one-size-fits-all approach. It is a personalized method that evolves with you as you learn to interpret and honor the signs and signals your body communicates. By doing so, you not only enhance your physical fitness but also foster a deeper connection with your body, leading to a more balanced and fulfilling lifestyle.

Chapter Summary

- The menstrual phase affects exercise routines; engaging in gentler workouts can be helpful due to low energy and strength from decreased estrogen and progesterone levels.
- Recommended activities during menstruation include gentle yoga, walking, swimming, and Pilates to accommodate the body's need for rest and recovery.
- During the follicular phase, rising estrogen levels lead to increased energy and pain tolerance, making it ideal for strength training and intense cardiovascular workouts
- The follicular phase is also an excellent time to focus on flexibility and balance, set new fitness goals, and try new activities while ensuring proper rest and nutrition.
- With a surge in hormones, the ovulatory phase is optimal for high-intensity and high-impact workouts, focusing on strength training and cardiovascular exercises.
- Group fitness and team sports can be enjoyable during the ovulatory phase, but it's essential to warm up properly and stay hydrated and nourished.
- In the luteal phase, rising progesterone may cause bloating and fatigue, so moderate-intensity activities like strength

- training with moderate weights and gentle yoga or Pilates are recommended.
- Listening to your body's unique signals throughout the cycle is crucial for tailoring workouts, with attention to physical, emotional, and mental cues, and journaling can aid in recognizing patterns.

4

CYCLE ALIGNMENT IN YOUR PERSONAL LIFE

Social Engagements and Your Cycle

Understanding the nuances of your menstrual cycle can be a transformative tool for organizing your social life. The concept of cycle alignment is not just limited to dietary adjustments or exercise routines; it extends into the realm of your social engagements, providing a useful framework for when to schedule activities, how to interact with others, and even how to manage your energy levels during various phases of your cycle.

During the follicular phase, which begins right after menstruation, your body is gearing up for potential conception. Estrogen levels are rising, leading to increased energy, brain function, and a more outgoing disposition. This is an excellent time to plan social outings, networking events, or any activity that requires active engagement and high energy. You may be more open to new experiences and meeting new people during this phase.

As you transition into the ovulatory phase, communication skills typically peak due to the high estrogen and luteinizing hormone levels. This is an excellent time to have meaningful conversations, attend social gatherings, or give presentations. Your charisma and articulacy are at their highest, making this the optimal time for activities that require verbal communication and social finesse.

The luteal phase, which follows ovulation, can be a bit more complex. In the early part of this phase, you may still enjoy the benefits of high energy and sociability. However, as you move closer to menstruation, your body begins to prepare for a potential pregnancy or to shed the uterine lining. Energy levels may wane, and you might feel more inclined to turn inward. This is a period when you might prefer smaller, more intimate gatherings or quiet evenings at home. It's also a time to be mindful of your emotional state, as some may experience heightened sensitivity or mood swings due to fluctuating hormone levels.

Finally, during menstruation, your body is in a state of release and renewal. Energy is typically at its lowest, and this is a time for rest and reflection. Limiting social engagements during this phase and giving yourself permission to say no to invitations is perfectly acceptable. Focus on self-care and activities that allow for rejuvenation. It's a time to listen to your body and honor its need for rest.

By aligning your social calendar with your menstrual cycle, you can harness the natural levels of your energy and emotions. This doesn't mean you must rigidly follow these guidelines; life is unpredictable, and flexibility is key. However, awareness of your cycle can empower you to make choices that enhance your mental well-being and social satisfaction. It's about working with your body, rather than against it, to create a harmonious balance in your personal life.

Sex and Intimacy: Syncing with Your Partner

Understanding and harmonizing with our menstrual cycle can be profoundly transformative in the realm of personal relationships, particularly with our intimate partners. Cycle synchronization applies not only to our social lives and self-care routines but also extends into the intimate sphere of sex and relationships. By aligning our awareness of the hormonal fluctuations throughout the menstrual cycle with our sexual and emotional needs, we can foster a deeper connection with our partners and enhance our overall well-being.

During the menstrual phase, when energy levels are lower and the body is going through a renewal process, it is natural for some to experience decreased libido. This is a time for open communication with your partner about your needs for comfort and support. Intimacy during this phase doesn't have to be solely about sexual activity; it can also be about cultivating closeness through gentle touch, warm embraces, or simply being in each other's presence.

As you transition into the follicular phase, your energy begins to rise, and so does your potential for sexual desire. This is an excellent time to engage in more active dates and explore new experiences together, both inside and outside the bedroom. The increase in estrogen makes this a prime time for emotional openness and trying new things, which can include experimenting with different forms of sexual expression.

The ovulatory phase often brings with it a peak in libido due to the surge in hormones like estrogen and testosterone. Communication can become more effortless, making you feel more connected to your partner. It's a time when many feel their most confident and expressive, making it an opportune moment to express desires and enjoy a heightened sense of intimacy.

Finally, during the luteal phase, as the body prepares for the possibility of pregnancy or the onset of the menstrual phase, some may experience premenstrual syndrome (PMS), which can affect mood and desire. During this time, remember to be patient with yourself and communicate any emotional or physical needs to your partner. This phase can be a time for deeper emotional bonding and nurturing intimacy in ways that are less physically demanding but equally fulfilling.

Sharing your cycle with your partner and discussing how it impacts your feelings and desires can create a shared understanding and a more empathetic approach to intimacy. It's not about adhering strictly to a schedule but about using the knowledge of your cycle to enhance communication and connection with your partner.

Remember, every individual's experience with their cycle is unique, and it's about finding what works best for you and your partner and using the understanding of your cycle as a tool to support each other's needs and deepen your bond.

Self-Care and Pampering Throughout the Cycle

In the journey of embracing cycle alignment, self-care and pampering are rewarding activities that can enhance your quality of life and fortify your connection with your body's natural rhythms. This practice of aligning self-care routines with the different phases of your menstrual cycle can be both a source of comfort and a tool for empowerment.

During the menstrual phase, when energy levels typically wane and the body calls for rest, it is essential to honor this inward pull. This is a time for gentle self-care. Consider warm baths infused with calming essential oils such as lavender or chamomile, which can soothe the body and the mind. Engage in restorative yoga or light stretching that honors your body's need for rest rather than pushing through high-intensity activities. Embrace the slower pace by curling up with a good book or practicing meditation and deep breathing exercises to center your thoughts and emotions.

As you transition into the follicular phase, your energy begins to rise. Capitalize on this increase by integrating more invigorating self-care practices. This might be the perfect time to try out a new fitness class or engage in creative activities that align with this phase's heightened mental clarity and enthusiasm. Pampering yourself could include a revitalizing facial or a massage that stimulates circulation, complementing the body's natural uptick in energy.

The ovulatory phase allows one to focus on self-care practices that foster connection and expression. This is when you might feel most social and communicative, so consider scheduling appointments for haircuts or beauty treatments that make you feel most confident and radiant. It's also an opportue moment to engage in activities that involve others, like group dance classes or social gatherings, which can be a form of self-care in their own right.

Finally, during the luteal phase, as the body prepares for the possibility of pregnancy or the onset of menstruation, you might experience more physical and emotional sensitivity. This is a time to be particularly gentle with yourself. Opt for self-care that grounds and stabilizes, such as a warm stone massage, acupuncture, or simply ensuring you have ample time for rest. Nutrition also plays a crucial role in self-care during this phase; focus on nourishing foods that support your body's needs, such as magnesium-rich leafy greens and complex carbohydrates, to help manage energy levels and mood.

Incorporating these tailored self-care practices into your routine not only honors your body's natural cycle but also reinforces a nurturing relationship with yourself. By listening to and respecting your body's signals, you create a foundation of well-being that supports you in all facets of life. Remember, the essence of cycle alignment in self-care is about making space for your needs and embracing your body's natural fluctuations with grace and kindness.

Emotional Well-being and Hormonal Fluctuations

The interplay between emotional well-being and hormonal fluctuations is highly relevant to understanding and fully reaping the benefits of cycle alignment. Our hormones are not just biological substances; they are the conductors of the orchestra that is our body, influencing our emotions, energy levels, and overall sense of well-being. We can harness our innate rhythms to foster emotional balance and resilience by tuning into these hormonal cues across our cycle.

During the menstrual phase, when both estrogen and progesterone are at their lowest, you might experience a sense of withdrawal or introspection. It's a time when some may feel more sensitive or prone to introspection. This is a natural period for reflection, and it's beneficial to allow yourself the space to process your emotions, perhaps by journaling or engaging in gentle, meditative activities.

As you transition into the follicular phase, estrogen rises, leading to an increase in energy and a more upbeat mood. The boost in confidence and creativity can be channeled into personal growth and exploration. This is an opportune time to tackle new projects and engage in social activities. Embrace this phase by setting intentions and goals, knowing your body is primed to support you in these endeavors.

The ovulatory phase is often marked by a peak in estrogen and the presence of luteinizing hormone, which can result in feeling more communicative and connected with others. It's a period where you might be more emotionally open and articulate. Leveraging this time for meaningful conversations and fostering relationships can be incredibly fruitful.

Finally, the luteal phase, which leads to menstruation, is characterized by higher progesterone levels. This shift can bring about a more reflective state and a tendency towards nesting and nurturing for some. It's not uncommon to experience premenstrual syndrome (PMS), where emotions can feel more intense or volatile. Recognizing these patterns allows you to plan for self-care strategies to mitigate stress and provide comfort.

By syncing your life with your cycle, you can anticipate and use these emotional shifts to your advantage. It's about creating a personal toolkit that aligns with your hormonal landscape—knowing when to push forward with vigor and when to pull back and replenish. This approach does not suggest that you are at the mercy of your hormones but rather that you can work with them to cultivate a harmonious balance in your emotional life.

Remember, every individual's experience with their cycle is unique. It's essential to observe your patterns and responses. Keeping a cycle diary can be invaluable in this process, helping you identify trends and tailor your approach to cycle syncing to support your emotional well-being best.

By embracing the wisdom of your body's natural rhythms, you can navigate the natural flow of your emotions with grace and self-compassion, leading to a more empowered and harmonious personal life.

Planning Personal Events and Activities by Cycle Phase

Cycle alignment emerges as a transformative approach to harmonize our personal lives with our natural rhythms. We can optimize our energy, productivity, and overall well-being by aligning our personal activities and events with the different phases of our menstrual cycle. This section will guide you through planning your events and activities according to the different phases of your cycle, ensuring that you are working with your body, not against it.

As we explored in earlier chapters, the menstrual phase is usually accompanied by lower energy levels due to the shedding of the uterine lining. It is a time for introspection and rest. This is an excellent opportunity to schedule low-key activities that do not demand high physical exertion, such as gentle yoga, meditation, or simply curling up with a good book. It's also a period for reflection, making it ideal for journaling or planning future goals.

As we transition into the follicular phase, our energy and estrogen levels rise. This is the time to tackle new projects and challenges. It's an excellent phase for brainstorming sessions, starting new hobbies, or planning outings that require more physical activity, such as hiking or cycling. The increase in energy and optimism makes it a favorable time to engage in social activities and network.

The ovulatory phase is often when energy peaks, alongside a surge in communication skills due to the high estrogen and testosterone levels. This is the prime time for important meetings, presentations, or any event where you need to be at your most articulate and charismatic. It's also a great time for social gatherings, parties, or date nights, as you'll likely feel more outgoing and connected.

Finally, the luteal phase, which leads up to menstruation, is characterized by a gradual decline in energy as the body prepares for the potential of pregnancy. This phase can be utilized for completing tasks, following up on projects, and wrapping up loose ends. It's also a period where some may experience premenstrual syndrome (PMS), so it's wise to avoid scheduling highly stressful events or demanding physical challenges. Instead, focus on activities that promote relaxation and self-care, such as a spa day or a creative endeavor that brings you joy.

By syncing your personal life with your cycle, you can create a rhythm that respects your body's natural fluctuations and empowers you to make the most of each phase. With this mindful approach, you can enhance your personal life, ensuring that you are living in a fulfilling and sustainable way.

Chapter Summary

- Cycle alignment can optimize social life by scheduling activities according to the menstrual cycle phases, enhancing energy management and interactions.
- The follicular phase is ideal for high-energy social outings and new experiences due to rising estrogen levels and increased outgoingness.
- The ovulatory phase is best for important conversations and social events, with peak communication skills and charisma due to high estrogen and luteinizing hormone levels.
- Early in the luteal phase can be suitable for socializing, but the latter part is better for intimate gatherings or solitude as energy wanes and mood may fluctuate.
- The menstrual phase is a time for rest and self-care, with reduced social activity and focus on rejuvenation as energy is at its lowest.
- Intimate relationships benefit from cycle syncing, with varying sexual and emotional needs throughout the cycle leading to deeper connections with partners.
- Self-care can be tailored to each cycle phase, with activities ranging from restorative practices during menstruation to energizing and social activities during ovulation.
- Planning your events and activities by cycle phase can enhance productivity and well-being, with each phase offering different opportunities for engagement and rest.
- Hormonal fluctuations influence emotional well-being, and understanding this can help manage emotions and foster resilience throughout the cycle.

5

CYCLE ALIGNMENT IN YOUR PROFESSIONAL LIFE

Productivity and Your Menstrual Cycle

Understanding the intricate relationship between your menstrual cycle and productivity can be a professional game-changer. Cycle synchronization is not just about physical health; it's about harnessing the rhythm of your hormonal landscape to optimize your work life. Let's delve into how the different phases of your menstrual cycle can impact your productivity and how you can leverage this knowledge to your advantage.

As we explored in previous chapters, each phase of the cycle comes with its own set of hormonal fluctuations that can influence your energy levels, cognitive functions, and overall work performance.

During the menstrual phase, when you typically experience lower energy levels, you may prefer to engage in less demanding tasks and introspection. This could be an opportune moment to reflect on your work goals, evaluate past performances, and plan ahead. While it might not be the time for aggressive brainstorming sessions or high-stakes negotiations, it's ideal for setting intentions and organizing tasks that require more focus and less physical exertion. Strategic thinking, long-term planning, and evaluating past performance can be done effectively during this time. It's also a period to be gentle with yourself, scheduling fewer meetings and allowing for more flexible deadlines when possible.

As you transition into the follicular phase, a rise in estrogen levels leads to increased energy, improved mood, and sharper cognitive abilities. This is the time to tackle challenging projects, brainstorm innovative ideas, and take on tasks that require more critical thinking and creativity. Your capacity for complex problem-solving is heightened, making it an excellent time for strategic planning and decision-making.

The ovulatory phase is often characterized by a peak in energy and communication skills, thanks to a surge in estrogen and testosterone. This is when you're likely to feel your most confident and articulate. Capitalize on this phase by scheduling important meetings, presentations, and networking events. It's a prime time for collaborative projects and initiatives that require teamwork and leadership.

Finally, during the luteal phase, you might find your focus turning inwards again, with a preference for completing tasks and tying up loose ends. This is a signal to switch gears from the high-energy tasks of the previous weeks to more detail-oriented and organizational activities. It's an excellent time to focus on completing tasks, following up on emails, and setting your agenda for the coming weeks. You may also find this is when you're best at critical analysis and editing work. While you may start to feel a dip in energy as this phase progresses, it's an opportune time to evaluate the outcomes of your efforts and prepare for the quieter, reflective period of the menstrual phase.

By acknowledging and adapting to the natural fluctuations of your menstrual cycle, you can create a work rhythm that not only respects your body's needs but also maximizes your professional potential. This approach to productivity is not about pushing through at all costs; it's about working smarter by aligning your tasks with the innate capabilities of each cycle phase. With this knowledge, you can craft a more harmonious and effective work life, one that empowers you to perform at your best while also honoring your body.

Communication and Collaboration During Different Phases

Understanding the intricacies of your menstrual cycle can be a powerful tool for enhancing communication and collaboration in the workplace. By aligning your professional interactions with the hormonal changes of your cycle, you can optimize your effectiveness and foster better relationships with colleagues.

During the menstrual phase, which marks the beginning of your cycle, you may experience a desire for introspection. This is a time for clear and concise communication. Prioritize essential conversations and allow yourself to listen more. You might find that your capacity for empathy is heightened during this phase, which can be leveraged to strengthen connections with coworkers. However, it can help to set boundaries to ensure you don't become overwhelmed.

As you transition into the follicular phase, your energy begins to rise, and so does your capacity for creative thinking and problem-solving. This is an opportune time to initiate new team projects and brainstorm with your colleagues. Your communication can become more assertive, and you may feel more inclined to lead discussions. Use this time to schedule meetings that require strategic planning and innovative thinking.

The ovulatory phase is often when you're most communicative and charismatic. Your ability to articulate ideas and your openness to collaboration are at their peak. This is the moment to tackle important negotiations, presentations, and networking opportunities. Embrace your persuasive skills and engage in team-building activities. Your natural magnetism during this phase can help inspire and motivate those around you.

Finally, during the luteal phase, as your body prepares for the possibility of pregnancy or the onset of the menstrual phase, you may notice a shift toward a more reflective state. While you may feel less inclined to socialize with others, you can use this time to provide thoughtful feedback and complete tasks that require focus and persistence. Communication may need to be more measured, as you might find yourself more sensitive to feedback or conflict.

By aligning your communication style and collaborative efforts with the natural fluctuations of your cycle, you can work more harmoniously with your biological rhythms and those around you. You can anticipate shifts in your capabilities and preferences, allowing you to approach tasks and interactions with intention.

Navigating workplace dynamics with cycle awareness is a powerful strategy for professional development. By understanding and working with the rhythms of your cycle, you can create a work life that is more productive and more harmonious with your natural rhythms. This holistic approach to professional growth respects your body's needs and career aspirations, leading to a more balanced and fulfilling work experience.

Chapter Summary

- Cycle alignment in the workplace involves aligning work tasks with the menstrual cycle phases to optimize productivity and professional potential.
- The menstrual phase is a time for introspection and planning, suitable for setting professional goals and organizing tasks requiring focus but less physical exertion.
- The follicular phase brings increased energy and cognitive abilities, ideal for tackling challenging projects, brainstorming, and strategic decision-making.
- The ovulatory phase peaks in energy and communication skills, making it the best time for important meetings, presentations, and collaborative projects.
- The luteal phase is excellent for inward focus, completing tasks, and detail-oriented work, with a gradual energy decline as the phase progresses.
- Communication and collaboration in the workplace can be enhanced by understanding and aligning with the hormonal changes of the menstrual cycle.

- Managing energy levels at work according to the menstrual cycle phases can lead to a healthier work-life balance and increased productivity.
- Navigating workplace dynamics with cycle awareness can improve task management, communication, and overall professional development.

6

CYCLE ALIGNMENT AND FERTILITY

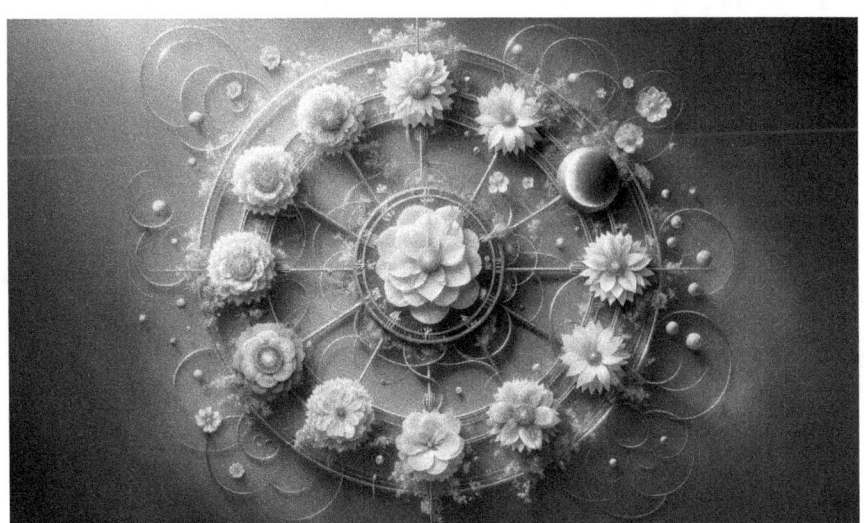

E mbarking on the journey of understanding fertility requires a comprehensive look at the menstrual cycle, a cornerstone of reproductive health. The menstrual cycle is not merely a timekeeper for potential conception; it is a barometer of overall well-being and a window into the intricate workings of the female body.

To grasp the concept of fertility within the cycle, one must first recognize that the menstrual cycle is divided into several phases and the role and contribution of each phase in fertility and contraception.

Ovulation is the pinnacle of fertility within the cycle. It is the moment when the mature egg is released from the ovary and is available for fertilization. The lifespan of the egg is relatively short, typically around 24 hours. Therefore, understanding the timing of ovulation is critical for those aiming to conceive or avoid pregnancy.

Tracking your menstrual cycle and recognizing the signs of each phase is a powerful tool for managing fertility. Body temperature, cervical mucus consistency, and hormonal changes are all indicators that can help pinpoint ovulation. Understanding these signs can help you build cycle alignment habits to optimize your health and achieve fertility goals.

Whether the aim is to enhance fertility or to use natural family planning methods for contraception, knowledge of your cycle is empowering. It allows for a harmonious relationship with the body's natural rhythms, fostering a sense of control and well-being. The next step in this journey is to delve into how cycle alignment can be applied to natural family planning, offering a practical approach to understanding and working with the body's fertility signals.

Natural Family Planning and Cycle Awareness

In understanding one's fertility, cycle awareness is a profound tool for natural family planning. This systematic approach to fertility awareness involves tracking the menstrual cycle to predict ovulation and plan or prevent pregnancy accordingly.

Cycle alignment for natural family planning is based on the principle that a woman is only fertile for a limited number of days during her cycle. By identifying these fertile days, couples can make informed decisions about when to engage in sexual activity, depending on their family planning goals.

The first step in natural family planning with cycle syncing is establishing a baseline understanding of your menstrual cycle. This requires regular observation and documentation over several months. You can record the start and end dates of your periods and any associated symptoms, such as cramping or mood changes, using the methods we discussed in earlier chapters.

Once you've identified your cycle pattern, you can shift your focus to pinpointing ovulation. Numerous physical signs can indicate the approach of ovulation, including changes in cervical mucus, a slight rise in basal body temperature, and even subtle shifts in libido or energy levels. You could also opt to use ovulation predictor kits for more precise identification of your fertile window.

During the fertile window, which typically spans five days leading up to and including the day of ovulation, couples seeking to conceive can increase their chances of pregnancy by having intercourse. Conversely, those who wish to avoid pregnancy can either abstain from sexual activity during this time or use barrier methods of contraception.

It's important to note that cycle syncing for natural family planning requires high commitment and self-awareness. Factors such as stress, illness, and lifestyle changes can all influence the menstrual cycle, potentially affecting the accuracy of fertility predictions. Therefore, paying close attention to your body and any factors that may cause variations in your cycle is beneficial.

This natural family planning method is most effective when cycles are regular and predictable. Women with irregular cycles may find it more challenging to use cycle alignment as a reliable form of natural family planning. They may need to explore additional methods or consult a healthcare professional for guidance.

Empowering yourself with the knowledge of cycle syncing for natural family planning fosters a deeper connection with your body. It provides a sense of control and partnership in the reproductive process. It is a natural, non-invasive approach that, when practiced diligently, can be a powerful ally in the journey of fertility management.

Optimizing Fertility Through Lifestyle Choices

Beyond the biological mechanics, lifestyle choices play a significant role in optimizing fertility. By aligning daily habits with the body's natural rhythms, you can create an environment conducive to conception.

Nutrition is a cornerstone of reproductive health. A diet rich in whole foods provides the necessary vitamins and minerals that support hormonal balance and egg quality. During the follicular phase, when the body is preparing for ovulation, incorporating foods high in antioxidants, such as berries and leafy greens, can aid in protecting the eggs from oxidative stress. As one transitions into the luteal phase, the focus shifts to foods that support progesterone production, like those rich in B vitamins and omega-3 fatty acids, found in whole grains and fatty fish, respectively.

Physical activity, too, should be tailored to the menstrual cycle. During the first half of the cycle, energy levels tend to be higher, making it a suitable time for more vigorous exercises, which can improve blood flow and reduce stress. As the cycle progresses, particularly after ovulation, gentler activities like yoga or walking can help maintain a sense of calm and reduce inflammation without overly taxing the body.

Stress management is another critical element. Chronic stress can disrupt the delicate hormonal interplay necessary for ovulation and implantation. Techniques such as mindfulness meditation, deep-breathing exercises, or engaging in hobbies that bring joy can mitigate stress and promote a more harmonious internal environment.

Sleep quality cannot be underestimated in its importance for fertility. Adequate, restorative sleep helps regulate the hormones that drive the menstrual cycle. Maintaining a consistent sleep schedule and creating a restful sleeping environment can bolster overall health and, by extension, fertility.

Lastly, environmental factors such as exposure to toxins should be minimized. Chemicals in certain plastics, personal care products, and household cleaners can have estrogen-like effects on the body, potentially disrupting hormonal balance. Opting for natural or organic alternatives can reduce this exposure and support the body's natural hormonal rhythms.

You can nurture your fertility by making conscious lifestyle choices that honor your body's cyclical nature. This holistic approach to health supports the physical dimension of conception and fosters a deeper connection with one's own body, empowering individuals on their path to parenthood.

Dealing with Infertility and Cycle Irregularities

Embarking on the journey to conceive can be filled with a spectrum of emotions, from excitement and hope to anxiety and uncertainty. When faced with infertility and cycle irregularities, these feelings can intensify. It's helpful to approach these challenges with a sense of empowerment and a systematic plan to navigate the complexities they present.

Infertility, commonly defined as the inability to conceive after one year of unprotected intercourse for women under 35 or after six months for women over 35, affects many couples worldwide. Cycle irregularities, manifesting as irregular periods, anovulation, or hormonal imbalances, can further complicate the ability to conceive. Understanding and addressing these issues cannot be missed in the journey towards conception.

Aligning lifestyle choices with the different phases of your menstrual cycle can be a valuable tool in managing infertility and cycle irregularities. By becoming attuned to the body's natural rhythms, you can implement targeted strategies that may enhance your fertility.

The first step in dealing with these challenges is to gather comprehensive information. This involves tracking menstrual cycles, noting the length, regularity, and symptoms experienced throughout. Apps and journals can be helpful tools in this process. A thorough understanding of your cycle provides invaluable insights and can help healthcare providers diagnose and treat any underlying issues.

Next, it's essential to seek professional guidance. A fertility specialist can conduct a range of tests to determine the cause of infertility or irregular cycles. These may include blood tests to assess hormone levels, ultrasounds to examine the reproductive organs and other diagnostic procedures. With this information, a tailored treatment plan can be developed, including cycle-syncing techniques, medical interventions, or a combination of both.

For those experiencing cycle irregularities, cycle alignment can be particularly beneficial. One can support hormonal balance and overall reproductive health by focusing on nutrition, exercise, stress management, and sleep patterns in accordance with the menstrual phases. For instance, when estrogen levels rise during the follicular phase, engaging in more intense physical activity and consuming a diet rich in phytoestrogens might be advantageous. Conversely, when progesterone is dominant during the luteal phase, emphasizing stress-reduction techniques and ensuring adequate intake of B vitamins could be more beneficial.

In addition to lifestyle modifications, medical treatments such as hormone therapy or assisted reproductive technologies (ART) may be necessary. These interventions should be considered part of a holistic approach, where cycle alignment plays a supportive role.

It's also important to acknowledge the emotional toll that infertility and cycle irregularities can take. Whether through counseling, support groups, or mindfulness practices, mental health support is a vital component of care. Emotional well-being is intrinsically linked to physical health, and nurturing both is paramount in creating the most supportive environment for conception.

In conclusion, while infertility and cycle irregularities present significant challenges, they are not insurmountable. With a proactive and informed approach, incorporating cycle alignment as a complementary practice and harnessing the expertise of healthcare professionals, individuals, and couples can enhance their fertility potential. By taking control of your health and making informed decisions, the path to parenthood, though sometimes winding, becomes clearer and more navigable.

Preconception Care and Cycle Alignment

Embarking on the journey to parenthood can be a time of great anticipation and, sometimes, anxiety.

Preconception care is a critical phase where potential parents can take proactive steps to enhance their health and well-being, creating the best possible environment for conception. Cycle alignment can be a valuable tool in this preparatory stage.

The menstrual cycle is a barometer of overall health, and its regularity often indicates a balanced hormonal environment. Observing and charting the menstrual cycle allows one to gain insights into their unique hormonal patterns and identify potential issues that could affect fertility. Cycle syncing empowers individuals to work with their bodies, rather than against them, by tailoring their preconception regimen to the natural rhythms of their cycle.

During the follicular phase, which begins after menstruation and leads up to ovulation, estrogen levels rise, and the body prepares for the possibility of pregnancy. This is when energy levels may increase, and the body is more receptive to nutrient-rich foods and moderate to high-intensity exercise. Emphasizing a diet rich in antioxidants, lean proteins, and complex carbohydrates can support egg health and hormonal balance.

As the cycle progresses to ovulation, this is the prime time for conception. Understanding the signs of ovulation, such as changes in cervical mucus and basal body temperature, can help in timing intercourse for the best chances of fertilization. Engaging in gentle stress-reduction techniques like yoga or meditation can also create a more conducive environment for conception.

Following ovulation, the luteal phase begins, marked by the production of progesterone, which prepares the uterine lining for potential implantation. During this phase, the body's basal metabolic rate increases, and additional calories may be needed. Choosing foods high in B vitamins and omega-3 fatty acids can support progesterone levels and reduce inflammation. Lighter exercise, such as walking or pilates, can maintain physical health without overly stressing the body.

In addition to dietary and exercise modifications, preconception care should also address other lifestyle factors that can impact fertility. This includes managing stress levels, as chronic stress can disrupt hormonal balance and menstrual regularity. Adequate sleep, mindfulness practices, and counseling or support groups can be beneficial in maintaining emotional equilibrium.

Environmental toxins are another consideration in preconception care. Exposure to certain chemicals in plastics, personal care products, and household cleaners can interfere with hormonal function. Adopting a more natural, organic lifestyle can reduce these exposures and support overall reproductive health.

Lastly, preconception care is not solely the responsibility of the individual trying to conceive. Partners can also engage in cycle alignment by being supportive and involved in lifestyle changes, understanding the menstrual cycle's phases, and contributing to a stress-free environment conducive to conception.

By integrating cycle syncing into preconception care, individuals and couples can feel empowered in their journey toward fertility. This practical approach allows for a deeper connection with one's body and can pave the way for a healthy pregnancy and beyond. It is a testament to the power of informed, proactive health management and the beauty of working in harmony with the body's natural processes.

Chapter Summary

- The menstrual cycle is a key indicator of reproductive health and overall well-being.
- Ovulation is the peak of fertility in the cycle, with a short egg lifespan, making timing knowledge crucial for conception or contraception.
- Tracking the menstrual cycle's signs, such as body temperature and cervical mucus, aids in cycle syncing to optimize health and fertility goals.
- Cycle syncing for natural family planning involves identifying fertile days to plan or prevent pregnancy, requiring careful cycle observation and documentation.
- Lifestyle choices, including diet and exercise tailored to the menstrual cycle, significantly optimize fertility.
- Infertility and cycle irregularities can be managed by cycle syncing, professional guidance, and possibly medical treatments, with attention to emotional well-being.

- Preconception care with cycle syncing involves aligning diet, exercise, and lifestyle with menstrual phases to prepare the body for pregnancy.
- Partners can support preconception care by understanding the menstrual cycle and contributing to a healthy environment for conception.

7

CYCLE ALIGNMENT FOR HEALTH CONDITIONS

PCOS and Cycle Alignment

Polycystic Ovary Syndrome, commonly known as PCOS, is a condition characterized by hormonal imbalances that can affect a woman's menstrual cycle, fertility, and various aspects of her health. Cycle alignment has emerged as a potential method to help manage the symptoms of PCOS.

In the follicular phase, which starts on the first day of menstruation and lasts until ovulation, women with PCOS may benefit from gentle, low-intensity exercises and focusing on foods that support estrogen production and balance blood sugar levels, including high-fiber foods, lean proteins, and omega-3 fatty acids.

As the cycle progresses into the ovulatory phase, it is often recommended to incorporate foods rich in B vitamins and zinc, which can support ovulation. Moderate-intensity exercises like cycling or swimming can be introduced, as they help boost energy levels and improve mood.

During the luteal phase, which occurs after ovulation and before the start of menstruation, women with PCOS may experience premenstrual syndrome (PMS) symptoms more intensely. To combat this, a diet rich in magnesium, calcium, and fiber can be helpful. These nutrients can be found in leafy greens, nuts, seeds, and whole grains. Stress management techniques, such as deep breathing exercises and mindfulness meditation, can also be beneficial during this time to help manage any mood swings or anxiety.

Finally, in the menstrual phase, focusing on hydration and replenishing iron levels due to blood loss is essential. Iron-rich foods such as lean meats, legumes, and spinach can be incorporated into the diet. Light exercise, such as stretching or restorative yoga, can help alleviate cramps and maintain circulation.

It is crucial to note that while cycle syncing can be a valuable tool for managing PCOS symptoms, it should be approached with individualized care and in consultation with a healthcare provider. Each woman's experience with PCOS is unique, and what works for one may not work for another. Therefore, a personalized approach that considers the individual's specific needs and symptoms is essential.

Moreover, cycle syncing is not a standalone treatment for PCOS. It is most effective when combined with other medical or therapeutic interventions recommended by healthcare professionals. This holistic approach can empower women with PCOS to take charge of their health and well-being, improving their quality of life and alleviating the symptoms associated with this condition.

Endometriosis and Menstrual Health

Endometriosis is a chronic condition that affects an estimated 1 in 10 women during their reproductive years. This condition is characterized by the presence of endometrial-like tissue outside the uterus, which can lead to a myriad of symptoms, including, but not limited to, severe menstrual pain, chronic pelvic pain, and infertility. The complexity of endometriosis and its impact on menstrual health calls for a multifaceted approach to management, one of which may include cycle alignment.

Understanding and adapting to the body's natural rhythms can be particularly empowering for women with endometriosis. It offers a sense of control over a condition that often feels unpredictable and unmanageable.

During the menstrual phase, when cramping and pain can be at their worst for those with endometriosis, a focus on anti-inflammatory foods and gentle movement can provide some relief. Foods rich in omega-3 fatty acids, such as flaxseeds and walnuts, and antioxidant-rich fruits and vegetables can help reduce inflammation. Gentle yoga or walking can maintain circulation and reduce discomfort without exacerbating symptoms.

Ovulation may present a unique set of challenges for those with endometriosis, as this is a time when symptoms can either improve or worsen. Listening to one's body and adjusting activities and diet is essential. Some may find they can maintain increased activity levels, while others may need to back up.

Finally, during the luteal phase, when premenstrual symptoms can mimic or exacerbate endometriosis pain, it's crucial to continue focusing on anti-inflammatory foods and incorporate stress-reduction techniques. Practices such as meditation, deep-breathing exercises, and restorative yoga can help manage stress, which can help regulate hormone levels and potentially reduce symptoms.

It's important to note that cycle syncing is not a cure for endometriosis but rather a complementary approach to help manage symptoms. Each woman's experience with endometriosis is unique, and what works for one may not work for another. Therefore, it's crucial to approach cycle syncing with a spirit of self-exploration and to work closely with healthcare providers to create a personalized plan that considers all aspects of health.

In addition to lifestyle modifications, medical treatments for endometriosis may include hormonal therapies, pain management strategies, and, in some cases, surgery. Cycle alignment can be integrated into a broader treatment plan, offering a holistic approach that empowers women to manage their condition actively.

By aligning lifestyle choices with the menstrual cycle, women with endometriosis can improve their quality of life and better understand their bodies. It's a journey of self-care that acknowledges the intricate connection between our daily habits and menstrual health.

Thyroid Health and Menstrual Regulation

Understanding the intricate dance between thyroid function and menstrual health is a pivotal step in harnessing the power of cycle alignment to manage and potentially improve various health conditions. The thyroid gland, a small butterfly-shaped organ located at the base of your neck, plays a crucial role in regulating metabolism, energy levels, and, importantly for our discussion, the menstrual cycle.

Thyroid hormones, primarily thyroxine (T4) and triiodothyronine (T3) influence the menstrual cycle by interacting with sex hormones. An imbalance in thyroid function can lead to menstrual irregularities such as amenorrhea (absence of menstruation), menorrhagia (heavy menstrual bleeding), or oligomenorrhea (infrequent menstruation). These conditions can be distressing and impact your quality of life, fertility, and overall health.

Cycle alignment can be particularly beneficial for those with thyroid-related menstrual irregularities. By understanding and working with the body's natural rhythms, it is possible to support thyroid health and, as a result, promote more regular menstrual cycles.

The follicular phase is an opportune time to focus on foods that support estrogen metabolism and thyroid function. Including foods rich in iodine, selenium, and zinc, such as seaweed, brazil nuts, and pumpkin seeds, can support thyroid hormone production and conversion.

As the body transitions into the ovulatory phase, the peak in estrogen can be leveraged to support thyroid health through moderate exercise, which can help maintain a healthy weight and reduce stress, both of which are beneficial for thyroid function.

During the luteal phase, some women may experience a slight dip in thyroid hormones. To counteract this, it can help to incorporate stress-reduction techniques such as yoga or meditation, as stress can exacerbate thyroid issues. Additionally, maintaining a consistent intake of complex carbohydrates during this phase can help stabilize blood sugar levels, which is important for both thyroid health and menstrual regularity.

It is important to note that while cycle alignment can be a powerful tool in managing thyroid health and menstrual regulation, it is not a substitute for medical treatment. Those with thyroid conditions such as hypothyroidism or hyperthyroidism should work closely with their healthcare provider to manage their condition, as medication may be necessary.

Incorporating cycle alignment into a holistic approach that includes medical treatment, when necessary, can empower women to take charge of their health. By understanding the interplay between the thyroid and menstrual cycle, women can make informed choices that support their well-being throughout the entire menstrual cycle.

As we explore the potential of cycle alignment for various health conditions, it becomes clear that awareness and personalization are key. Just as each woman's cycle is unique, so is how her body will respond to different phases and the strategies she can employ to support her health. With this knowledge, we can move forward to address premenstrual syndrome (PMS) and premenstrual dysphoric disorder (PMDD). These conditions also benefit from a deeper understanding of the menstrual cycle and its connection to overall health.

Managing PMS and PMDD with Cycle Awareness

Premenstrual Syndrome (PMS) and Premenstrual Dysphoric Disorder (PMDD) are two health conditions that can significantly impact a woman's quality of life. While PMS is more common and its symptoms are typically milder, PMDD is a severe form of PMS that can be debilitating. Both conditions manifest in the luteal phase of the menstrual cycle, which is the period after ovulation and before the start of menstruation. Cycle alignment can be a powerful tool in managing the symptoms of PMS and PMDD.

Understanding the hormonal fluctuations that characterize the menstrual cycle is the first step in cycle syncing for PMS and PMDD. During the luteal phase, estrogen levels decline while progesterone levels rise and fall if pregnancy does not occur. It is these hormonal shifts that are thought to trigger the symptoms of PMS and PMDD. Symptoms can range from mood swings, bloating, and breast tenderness to more severe psychological symptoms such as anxiety and depression in the case of PMDD.

By becoming cycle-aware, women can anticipate the onset of these symptoms and implement strategies to mitigate them. For instance, dietary adjustments can play a significant role in symptom management. Focusing on foods rich in B vitamins, calcium, magnesium, and omega-3 fatty acids during the luteal phase can help alleviate mood swings and physical discomfort. Additionally, reducing the intake of caffeine, alcohol, and high-sodium foods may decrease bloating and fluid retention.

Stress management techniques are also crucial during this phase. Practices such as mindfulness meditation, deep-breathing exercises, and journaling can help manage the emotional symptoms associated with PMS and PMDD. Sleep hygiene is equally important; adequate rest can help regulate mood and improve overall well-being.

For those with PMDD, where symptoms are more severe and disruptive, it may be necessary to work with a healthcare provider to develop a comprehensive treatment plan. This plan could include cycle alignment strategies and other interventions such as cognitive-behavioral therapy or medication.

In conclusion, cycle synchronization offers a proactive approach to managing the symptoms of PMS and PMDD. By understanding and working with the body's natural rhythms, women can empower themselves to take control of their well-being. It is a systematic and personalized strategy that can be adjusted as needed, providing a sense of agency over one's health. As we move forward, we will explore how stress, which can be both a trigger and an amplifier of menstrual symptoms, interacts with the menstrual cycle and what strategies you can use to mitigate its effects.

The Impact of Stress on Your Menstrual Cycle

To understand how various factors influence menstrual health, it is crucial to address the role of stress, a pervasive element in modern life that can significantly affect your menstrual cycle. Stress, whether acute or chronic, can disrupt the delicate hormonal balance that regulates the menstrual cycle, leading to a range of symptoms and conditions that may compromise overall well-being.

The menstrual cycle is orchestrated by a symphony of hormones, primarily estrogen and progesterone, sensitive to stress-induced changes. When you experience stress, your body produces higher cortisol levels, a hormone released by the adrenal glands. Cortisol is often called the "stress hormone" because it helps your body manage and adapt to stress. However, when cortisol levels are consistently elevated, it can lead to a hormonal imbalance, affecting the production and regulation of reproductive hormones.

This hormonal disruption can manifest in various ways. For some, it may cause irregularities in the menstrual cycle, such as missed periods or unpredictable menstrual flow. For others, stress can exacerbate premenstrual symptoms, making the days leading up to menstruation particularly challenging. In more severe cases, chronic stress can contribute to the development of conditions such as amenorrhea and the absence of menstruation or can worsen the symptoms of polycystic ovary syndrome (PCOS).

Understanding the impact of stress on your menstrual cycle is the first step towards mitigating its effects. By recognizing the times when you may be more vulnerable to stress, you can implement strategies to bolster resilience and maintain hormonal balance.

During the follicular phase, when estrogen levels are rising, you may be more capable of handling stress due to the uplifting effects of this hormone. Conversely, when progesterone is dominant during the luteal phase, you may feel more inclined towards introspection and rest. Honoring these natural rhythms by adjusting your workload and stress management techniques can help maintain hormonal equilibrium.

Practical stress-reduction strategies include mindfulness meditation, deep-breathing exercises, regular physical activity, and ensuring adequate sleep. Nutrition is also pivotal in managing stress and supporting the menstrual cycle. A balanced diet rich in whole foods, emphasizing magnesium, vitamin B6, and omega-3 fatty acids, can provide the necessary nutrients to support your body's stress response and hormonal health.

By acknowledging the profound impact of stress on the menstrual cycle and adopting cycle alignment as a proactive approach to wellness, you can create a supportive environment for your body to thrive. This helps manage stress-related menstrual irregularities and empowers you to harness your body's innate wisdom, leading to improved health outcomes and a greater sense of harmony with your natural cycles.

Chapter Summary

- The symptoms of health conditions such as PCOS and endometriosis can be managed with cycle alignment, tailoring diet and exercise to menstrual phases, starting with estrogen-supportive foods and gentle exercise in the follicular phase.
- Thyroid health and menstrual regulation can benefit from cycle alignment, focusing on supporting thyroid function through diet and stress management across different menstrual phases.
- Managing symptoms of PMS and PMDD involves cycle awareness, dietary adjustments, tailored exercise, stress management, and possibly medical interventions for severe cases.
- Stress, whether acute or chronic, can disrupt the delicate hormonal balance that regulates your menstrual cycle and lead to a range of symptoms and conditions that may compromise your well-being.
- Acknowledging the profound impact of stress on the menstrual cycle and adopting cycle alignment as a proactive approach to wellness can help you create a supportive environment for your body to thrive.

8

HOLISTIC APPROACHES TO CYCLE ALIGNMENT

Integrating Mindfulness and Meditation

In the journey toward harmonizing with our body's natural rhythms, mindfulness, and meditation emerge as powerful tools for cycle syncing. These practices offer a pathway to deeper self-awareness and can significantly enhance our connection to the ebbs and flows of our menstrual cycle.

At its core, mindfulness is the practice of being fully present and engaged in the moment, aware of our thoughts and feelings without distraction or judgment. When applied to cycle syncing, mindfulness encourages us to tune into our body's signals and recognize the subtle shifts that occur throughout the different phases of our menstrual cycle. By observing these changes with a non-judgmental attitude, we can better understand our patterns and respond to our body's needs with compassion and care.

Meditation, a complementary practice to mindfulness, involves sitting quietly and focusing the mind, often on a particular object, thought, or activity, to achieve mental clarity and emotional calmness. During the menstrual cycle, meditation can be tailored to address the specific needs of each phase. For instance, during the menstrual phase, when energy may be lower, a guided visualization focused on rest and renewal can be particularly soothing. Conversely, when energy levels are typically higher during the ovulatory phase, a meditation centered on empowerment and creativity can help harness this vibrant energy.

Integrating mindfulness and meditation into cycle syncing not only aids in managing physical symptoms but also supports emotional well-being. It can help alleviate stress, which disrupts hormonal balance and promotes a sense of peace and grounding. This, in turn, can lead to more balanced cycles and a more profound sense of harmony with one's body.

To begin incorporating these practices, you could start with a simple daily mindfulness exercise, such as paying attention to your breathing or conducting a body scan to notice any areas of tension or ease. This can be done at any time of day and adjusted to fit into your schedule. Meditation can also be introduced gradually, with five to ten-minute sessions focusing on themes relevant to the current menstrual phase.

As we delve deeper into the holistic approaches to cycle syncing, it becomes evident that nurturing our menstrual health extends beyond the realm of the mind. The natural world offers a bounty of herbal remedies that have been used for centuries to support women's health. In the following discussion, we will explore how these herbal allies can be integrated into a holistic strategy for menstrual wellness, complementing the mindful practices of meditation and cycle awareness.

Herbal Remedies and Menstrual Health

Many individuals are turning toward the wisdom of herbal remedies to achieve a harmonious relationship with one's menstrual cycle. This ancient practice, deeply rooted in the knowledge of natural healers and traditional medicine, offers many options for those seeking to support their menstrual health through cycle syncing.

Herbs have been used for centuries to address various health issues, including those related to the menstrual cycle. Their application in cycle syncing is based on the understanding that different menstrual cycle phases may benefit from specific herbal support to optimize overall well-being.

During the follicular phase, the body is preparing for the possibility of ovulation and pregnancy. Herbs that support estrogen production and follicle growth can be particularly beneficial during this time. For example, Vitex agnus-castus, commonly known as chasteberry, is often recommended to help regulate hormonal imbalances and promote a healthy menstrual cycle.

As the cycle progresses into the ovulatory phase, the focus shifts to herbs that support the luteinizing hormone surge and the release of the egg. Herbs like Shatavari (Asparagus racemosus) and Evening Primrose Oil are known for their supportive role in enhancing fertility and maintaining hormonal balance.

The luteal phase, which follows ovulation, is when the body prepares for the potential of pregnancy or transitions into the menstrual phase. During this phase, herbs that support progesterone levels are key. For instance, Cimicifuga racemosa, also known as black cohosh, has been traditionally used to ease premenstrual symptoms and support the cycle's luteal phase.

Finally, during menstruation, the body benefits from herbs that can help alleviate cramps, regulate blood flow, and soothe the system. Ginger (Zingiber officinale) and Cramp Bark (Viburnum opulus) are two such herbs that have been revered for their effectiveness in reducing menstrual discomfort and supporting a healthy menstrual flow.

It is important to approach herbal remedies with an understanding of their potency and potential interactions with other medications. Consulting with a healthcare provider, particularly one specializing in herbal medicine or naturopathy, is essential before integrating these remedies into one's cycle alignment routine. This ensures personalized advice that considers individual health histories and current conditions.

Moreover, the quality of herbal supplements is paramount. Sourcing herbs from reputable suppliers and opting for organic, non-GMO options whenever possible can significantly enhance their therapeutic benefits. Attention to preparation and dosage is also crucial, as the efficacy of herbal remedies can vary greatly depending on these factors.

Incorporating herbal remedies into cycle alignment is not merely about addressing symptoms; it is about nurturing the body's natural rhythms and fostering a deeper connection with one's cyclical nature. By mindfully selecting and utilizing herbs that resonate with the different phases of the menstrual cycle, individuals can empower themselves to support their menstrual health in a holistic and nurturing manner.

As we explore holistic approaches to cycle alignment, the integration of various modalities becomes apparent. The next step in this journey delves into the ancient practice of Acupuncture and Traditional Chinese Medicine, which offers another layer of depth to understanding and supporting menstrual health.

Acupuncture and Traditional Chinese Medicine

In holistic health, acupuncture and Traditional Chinese Medicine (TCM) are time-honored practices with a rich tapestry of methods for addressing various health concerns, including menstrual health and cycle alignment. These ancient modalities offer a unique perspective on the body's energetic balance and provide tools for aligning one's cycle with the body's natural rhythms.

Acupuncture, a key component of TCM, involves the insertion of fine needles into specific points on the body to stimulate the flow of Qi or vital energy. According to TCM theory, the menstrual cycle is governed by the ebb and flow of this energy and the balance of the Yin and Yang forces within the body. By targeting acupuncture points linked to the reproductive organs, practitioners aim to harmonize these forces and promote a regular, pain-free menstrual cycle.

For those seeking to sync their cycles with their lifestyles, acupuncture can be particularly beneficial during different menstrual cycle phases. During the menstrual phase, for instance, acupuncture may focus on points that help to alleviate cramps and regulate blood flow. In the follicular phase, treatments aim to enhance energy levels and support the growth of the uterine lining. The ovulatory phase may emphasize points that encourage ovulation and fertility. In contrast, the luteal phase treatments could target points to alleviate symptoms of premenstrual syndrome (PMS) and support the potential early stages of pregnancy.

Beyond acupuncture, TCM also encompasses a holistic view of diet and lifestyle, advocating for a diet that supports menstrual health. Foods are chosen based on their energetic properties and ability to nourish the blood, support the Qi, and maintain the balance of Yin and Yang. For example, during the menstrual phase, it is suggested to consume warm, iron-rich foods to replenish lost blood and energy. In contrast, foods that support liver and kidney function, which are believed to be closely tied to reproductive health, are emphasized during the ovulatory phase.

Additionally, TCM practitioners may recommend specific exercises and practices that align with the energetic qualities of each menstrual phase. Gentle movements and breathing exercises can help maintain Qi's smooth flow throughout the body, which is essential for a balanced cycle.

It is important to note that while acupuncture and TCM offer a holistic approach to cycle syncing, they should be pursued with the guidance of a qualified practitioner. This ensures the treatments are tailored to the individual's unique constitution and health needs. Moreover, it is advisable to integrate these practices with conventional medical advice, particularly for those with underlying health conditions or those who are taking medications.

In summary, acupuncture and Traditional Chinese Medicine provide a comprehensive framework for understanding and nurturing menstrual health through cycle alignment. By considering the body's energetic landscape and employing targeted interventions, these practices aim to foster a harmonious menstrual cycle that resonates with the body's innate wisdom and the individual's lifestyle.

Yoga and Cycle Syncing

In the pursuit of aligning one's lifestyle with the intricacies of the menstrual cycle, yoga emerges as a potent ally. This ancient practice, rooted in the harmonization of body and mind, offers a dynamic approach to cycle syncing that can be tailored to the shifting phases of the menstrual cycle. By understanding the unique needs of each phase, individuals can employ specific yoga practices to support hormonal balance and overall well-being.

During the menstrual phase, when energy levels may be at their lowest, restorative yoga poses can be particularly beneficial. Gentle postures such as Supported Child's Pose, Reclining Bound Angle Pose, and Legs-Up-The-Wall encourage relaxation and help alleviate discomfort. Focusing on deep breathing and mindfulness during these poses also aids in reducing stress, which is crucial as stress hormones can exacerbate menstrual symptoms.

As you transition into the follicular phase, energy levels typically rise. This is an excellent time to engage in more dynamic and invigorating yoga sequences. Poses that promote strength and flexibility, such as Warrior II, Triangle Pose, and Sun Salutations, can be integrated to harness the body's growing vitality. This phase is also ideal for incorporating breathwork, or pranayama, techniques that enhance focus and invigorate the body, preparing it for the ovulatory phase.

The ovulatory phase, characterized by peak fertility and often the highest energy levels, allows for the exploration of more challenging poses and peak expressions. Balancing poses like Half Moon Pose or inversions such as Headstand can be practiced to take advantage of the body's full potential during this time. These poses not only build physical strength but also foster a sense of inner confidence and outward expressiveness.

Finally, during the luteal phase, energy may begin to wane as the body prepares for the possibility of pregnancy or the onset of menstruation. This is a period to honor the body's need for slowing down. Transitioning to a gentler practice focusing on hip-opening poses like Pigeon Pose and grounding postures such as Wide-Legged Forward Bend can support the body's natural processes. Additionally, incorporating cooling pranayama techniques can help soothe any premenstrual tension.

Incorporating yoga into cycle alignment is not merely about selecting appropriate poses for each phase but cultivating an intimate dialogue with your body. It requires attentiveness to your body's signals and a willingness to adapt one's practice to the ebb and flow of hormonal changes. By doing so, yoga becomes more than a physical exercise; it transforms into a holistic practice that nurtures the cyclical nature of the female body.

As we delve deeper into the holistic approaches to cycle syncing, it becomes evident that the interplay between various lifestyle factors is key to achieving hormonal harmony. The subsequent discussion will explore another pivotal aspect of this equilibrium: the role of sleep in hormonal balance. By understanding how sleep patterns can be optimized to support the menstrual cycle, you can further enhance your cycle synchronization efforts, leading to a more profound sense of health and vitality.

The Role of Sleep in Hormonal Balance

In the pursuit of achieving hormonal harmony, the significance of sleep cannot be overstated. As we delve into the intricacies of cycle alignment, it becomes clear that the quality and quantity of our slumber play a pivotal role in regulating our endocrine system. The circadian rhythm, an internal clock governing the sleep-wake cycle, is deeply intertwined with the ebb and flow of hormonal levels throughout the menstrual cycle.

The menstrual cycle is a complex interplay of hormones, primarily estrogen and progesterone, which fluctuate naturally. These fluctuations can influence sleep patterns, and conversely, sleep can affect the balance of these hormones. During the follicular phase, rising estrogen levels promote more restful sleep. In contrast, the luteal phase, characterized by higher progesterone levels, may disrupt sleep or lead to fatigue during the day.

Understanding this bidirectional relationship offers a powerful tool for women seeking to align their lifestyles with their biological rhythms. One can foster an environment conducive to hormonal equilibrium by prioritizing sleep hygiene. This involves establishing a consistent sleep schedule, optimizing the sleep environment for comfort and tranquility, and engaging in relaxing pre-sleep routines.

Moreover, the quality of sleep is just as important as its duration. Deep sleep stages are particularly restorative for the body and mind, allowing for the repair of tissues and the consolidation of memories. These stages also contribute to the regulation of cortisol, the stress hormone, which, when imbalanced, can have a cascading effect on other hormones.

To enhance sleep quality, limiting exposure to blue light from screens before bedtime is advisable, as it can interfere with the production of melatonin, the hormone responsible for inducing sleep. Additionally, dietary choices can have an impact; for instance, consuming caffeine or heavy meals too close to bedtime may hinder the ability to fall asleep or stay asleep.

Consider tailoring your evening activities and sleep environment to your menstrual cycle phase. For example, during the luteal phase, when sleep disturbances are more common, it may be beneficial to incorporate relaxation techniques such as meditation or gentle stretching before bed to promote better sleep quality.

By integrating sleep into the broader framework of cycle alignment, you can take proactive steps toward nurturing your hormonal health. This holistic approach enhances overall well-being and empowers you to live in greater synchrony with your body's natural rhythms. Through the strategic alignment of lifestyle choices with the menstrual cycle, you can unlock the full potential of your physical and emotional health, paving the way for a more balanced and fulfilling life.

Chapter Summary

- Mindfulness and meditation are key practices for syncing with the body's natural menstrual cycle, enhancing self-awareness and connection to the body's rhythms.
- Mindfulness involves being present and aware of bodily signals and changes during the menstrual cycle, while meditation can be tailored to the energy levels of each phase.
- These practices can help manage physical symptoms, reduce stress, and promote emotional well-being, leading to more balanced cycles.
- Simple mindfulness exercises like breath awareness or body scans can be incorporated daily, and meditation can start with short sessions focusing on themes relevant to the menstrual phase.

- Herbal remedies have been used for centuries to support menstrual health, with specific herbs beneficial for different phases of the menstrual cycle.
- Consulting with healthcare providers is crucial before using herbal remedies to ensure they are appropriate and to avoid interactions with other medications.
- Acupuncture and Traditional Chinese Medicine offer a holistic approach to cycle syncing, with acupuncture points targeted to balance the body's energy and support menstrual health.
- Yoga practices can be adapted to the menstrual cycle's phases, using restorative poses during menstruation and more active poses during other phases to support hormonal balance and well-being.
- Sleep plays a critical role in hormonal balance, with sleep patterns and menstrual cycle hormones influencing each other.
- Good sleep hygiene and understanding the relationship between sleep and hormonal fluctuations can help align lifestyle with biological rhythms for better health.

9

CREATING YOUR PERSONAL CYCLE ALIGNMENT PLAN

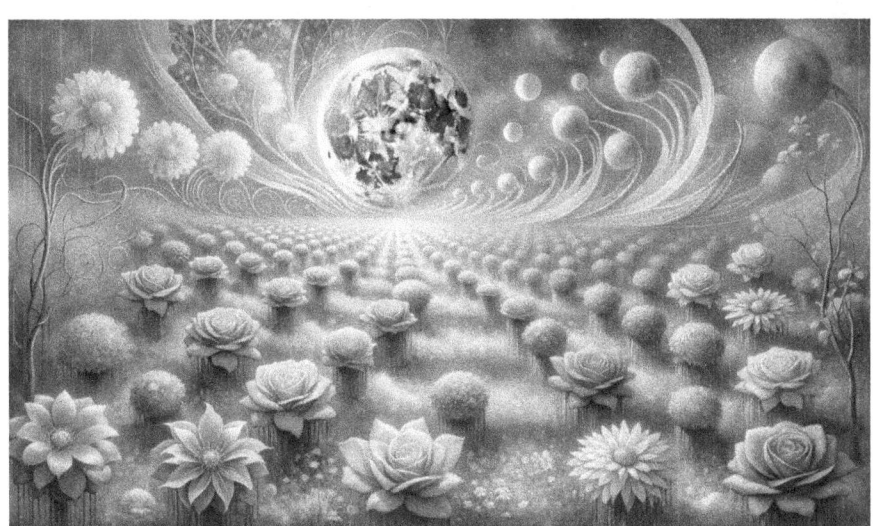

Embarking on the journey of cycle alignment requires a thoughtful assessment of your current lifestyle and menstrual cycle. This process is not about judgment or criticism; it's about understanding your unique rhythms and how they interact with your daily life. By evaluating your current situation, you can create a personalized plan that aligns with your body's natural cycles and supports your overall well-being.

Begin by tracking your menstrual cycle if you haven't already. This is the cornerstone of cycle syncing. Note your period's start and end dates, any symptoms you experience, and how you feel emotionally and physically throughout the different phases.

Next, take a candid look at your current lifestyle. How do your daily activities, work demands, social engagements, and exercise routines align with the different phases of your cycle? Are there times when you feel in sync with your body's needs and times when you don't? For instance, you might notice that high-intensity workouts feel more challenging during your menstrual phase or that you're more sociable and articulate during your ovulatory phase.

Consider also your nutrition. Are you fueling your body with the nutrients it needs to thrive throughout each phase of your cycle? Different phases may benefit from different dietary focuses, such as iron-rich foods during menstruation or more carbohydrates during the luteal phase to support energy levels.

Sleep patterns are another critical aspect to assess. Hormonal shifts throughout your cycle can impact your sleep quality and needs. Pay attention to any changes in your sleep patterns and how they correlate with the different phases of your cycle.

Stress levels and how you manage them should also be evaluated. Chronic stress can disrupt hormonal balance and affect your menstrual cycle. Reflect on the stressors in your life and how you might better manage them to support your hormonal health.

By conducting this comprehensive assessment, you are laying the groundwork for a cycle syncing plan tailored to your body's needs. This personalized approach will help you feel more in tune with your natural rhythms and empower you to make choices that enhance your health and vitality.

With this understanding of your current lifestyle and cycle, you are now ready to set goals and intentions to guide you in making the most of each phase of your cycle. This proactive step will ensure that your cycle syncing plan is well-informed and purpose-driven, setting you up for success in harmonizing your lifestyle with your body's innate patterns.

Setting Goals and Intentions

Embarking on the journey of cycle alignment is akin to setting sail on a voyage of self-discovery and holistic well-being. As you stand at the helm, ready to navigate the waters of your menstrual cycle with newfound knowledge and awareness, it is essential to chart a course that resonates with your aspirations and life circumstances. This voyage begins with setting goals and intentions, which will serve as your guiding stars throughout this transformative process.

Goals and intentions are more than mere wishes; they are the seeds from which the fruits of your efforts will grow. To set them effectively, you must reflect on what you hope to achieve through cycle syncing. You may seek to alleviate physical discomfort, enhance your emotional well-being, or optimize your productivity and creativity. Maybe you aim to deepen your connection with your body's natural rhythms or foster balance and harmony in your daily life. Whatever your desires may be, it is important to articulate them clearly and ensure they align with your core values and lifestyle.

When setting your goals, specificity is your ally. Rather than vague aspirations, define concrete objectives that can be measured and tracked. For instance, if your goal is to reduce premenstrual syndrome (PMS) symptoms, identify which symptoms you wish to address and what improvement would look like. If enhancing your productivity is your aim, determine what that means in the context of your work or personal projects. By being specific, you create a tangible target to aim for, making it easier to recognize progress and maintain motivation.

In addition to setting goals, it is equally important to establish intentions. While goals are the destinations you strive to reach, intentions are the attitudes and mindsets with which you approach your journey. They are the compass that keeps you oriented towards your true north, even when the seas become rough. Intentions could include cultivating patience with your body's processes, practicing self-compassion, or maintaining a sense of curiosity and openness to learning.

As you set your intentions, consider the following questions: How do you want to feel throughout your cycle? What personal strengths can you draw upon to support your goals? What mindset shifts might be necessary to embrace the ebbs and flows of your cycle? By answering these questions, you can craft intentions that not only complement your goals but also empower you to approach each phase of your cycle with grace and resilience.

Remember, setting goals and intentions is not a one-time event but an ongoing dialogue with yourself. As you progress in your cycle alignment journey, revisit and refine your goals and intentions to reflect your growth and any new insights you gain. This iterative process ensures that your cycle alignment plan remains dynamic and responsive to your evolving needs.

With your goals and intentions now clearly defined, you are well-prepared to move forward with designing your personalized cycle alignment strategy. This strategy will be your roadmap, detailing the practical steps you will take to align your daily life with the natural rhythms of your menstrual cycle. Here, the seeds of your goals and intentions will take root, and with careful nurturing, they will grow into a life that is in harmonious sync with your body's innate wisdom.

Designing Your Personalized Cycle Alignment Strategy

With your goals and intentions clearly outlined, it's time to move forward into the heart of cycle synchronization: designing your personalized strategy. This process is akin to crafting a tailored wellness plan that aligns with the unique rhythms of your body. It's about creating harmony between your lifestyle and your menstrual cycle, allowing you to harness the ebb and flow of your hormonal landscape.

Let's focus on the four distinct phases of your menstrual cycle: the menstrual phase, the follicular phase, the ovulatory phase, and the luteal phase. Each of these phases comes with its own hormonal fluctuations that can influence your energy levels, mood, and overall well-being.

Understanding these phases is the foundation upon which you will build your cycle-syncing strategy. Here's a summary of some of the strategies we covered in previous chapters:

- **Menstrual Phase:** During this time, when your energy may be at its lowest, consider gentle activities such as yoga, meditation, or light walking. Nutritionally, support your body with warm, nourishing foods rich in iron and protein to replenish what is lost during menstruation.
- **Follicular Phase:** As your energy rises, this is an opportune time to tackle new projects and engage in more vigorous exercise. Your diet can shift to include more raw foods and lighter fare that align with your body's increasing momentum.
- **Ovulatory Phase:** With energy typically at its peak, capitalize on this by scheduling important meetings or social engagements. High-impact workouts can be most beneficial during this phase. Foods rich in fiber can help support the body's natural detoxification processes.
- **Luteal Phase:** As you wind down, it's vital to start slowing your pace. Focus on completing tasks rather than starting new ones. Gentle exercise like swimming or cycling can be soothing. Cravings might arise; balance them with healthy fats and complex carbohydrates to maintain stable blood sugar levels.

Now, let's consider the personalization of your strategy. Start by tracking your cycle, if you aren't already, to pinpoint the length and particularities of each phase for you. This isn't a one-size-fits-all approach; your cycle is unique, and your plan should reflect that.

Next, integrate your goals and intentions. If you aim for improved fitness, align your workout intensity with the natural fluctuations in your energy. For career-focused goals, schedule demanding tasks during your follicular and ovulatory phases when you're likely to feel more outgoing and assertive.

Remember, this strategy should enhance your life, not complicate it.

Flexibility is key. If a high-energy activity is planned, but you're not feeling up to it, it's okay to adjust. Listening to your body is paramount; the goal is to sync with your cycle, not to be ruled by it.

As you design your plan, consider all aspects of your life—work, relationships, personal growth, and rest. Each should ebb and flow with your cycle, allowing you to optimize your time and energy effectively.

In the next section, we'll delve into implementing your plan, ensuring it fits seamlessly into your lifestyle, and making adjustments as needed. Remember, cycle syncing is a dynamic process, and your strategy should evolve with you as you gain insights and experience with your body's rhythms.

Implementing and Adjusting Your Plan

Having designed your personalized cycle syncing strategy, you are poised to embark on a transformative journey. Implementing your plan is a dynamic process that requires patience, observation, and the willingness to adapt. As you step into this phase, remember that your body's responses are unique, and your plan should be as fluid as the cycles you aim to sync with.

Begin by integrating the elements of your cycle-syncing strategy into your daily routine. This might involve adjusting your diet, exercise regimen, social engagements, and work tasks to align with the different phases of your menstrual cycle. For instance, when energy levels typically rise during the follicular phase, you might schedule more demanding projects or start new initiatives. Conversely, during the luteal phase, when you feel more introspective, you could plan for tasks requiring less social interaction and more detail-oriented work.

As you implement these changes, it's crucial to maintain a non-judgmental attitude towards yourself. Some days will be easier than others, and that's perfectly normal. The goal is not to achieve perfection but to cultivate a deeper understanding and harmony with your body's natural rhythms.

Monitoring your body's reactions to these adjustments is vital. You may find that certain assumptions you made during the planning stage don't hold true in practice. Perhaps a particular type of exercise you thought would be energizing during one phase of your cycle leaves you feeling depleted. Or you may discover that you're more social during the luteal phase than anticipated. These insights are valuable and should be used to refine your plan.

Adjusting your plan is not a sign of failure; it is a sign of attunement. It means you are listening to your body and respecting its signals. Make small, incremental changes rather than sweeping overhauls to avoid overwhelming yourself and observe the effect of each adjustment better.

Remember, the ultimate aim of cycle synchronization is to enhance your well-being and empower you to live in sync with your body's natural rhythms. This process is inherently personal and will evolve over time. Embrace the learning curve and allow your cycle alignment plan to be a living document that grows and changes as you do.

As you continue implementing and adjusting your plan, you'll gather valuable data about your body and its cycles. This data will be the foundation for the next step in your journey: tracking progress and making data-driven decisions, which will further refine your approach to cycle syncing and help you achieve the balance and harmony you seek.

Tracking Progress and Making Data-Driven Decisions

Remember to recognize that this is not a static plan but a dynamic process that evolves with you. The key to harnessing the full potential of cycle alignment lies in meticulously tracking your progress and making informed decisions based on the data you collect. This approach ensures that your personal cycle alignment plan is not only tailored to your unique rhythms but also adaptable to the changes your body may experience over time.

Begin by establishing a baseline. Document your physical, emotional, and mental states daily. Note your energy levels, mood fluctuations, sleep quality, dietary cravings, and physical symptoms. Utilize a journal or a digital tracking tool designed for cycle syncing to streamline this process. The objective is to gather enough data to discern patterns that correlate with the different phases of your menstrual cycle.

As you collect data, you'll start to notice trends. You may see that your energy peaks during the ovulatory phase or requires more rest during the luteal phase. These insights are invaluable as they guide you in fine-tuning your cycle syncing plan. For instance, you may schedule demanding tasks when your energy is naturally higher or incorporate more self-care practices when you need additional rest.

Pay attention to the outliers – days when you don't feel as expected based on your cycle phase. These instances can be just as informative, prompting you to consider external factors such as stress, diet, or exercise that may influence your well-being. Acknowledging these variables allows you to adjust your plan to support your body's needs better.

Remember, tracking aims not to judge or critique your experiences but to understand them. This understanding empowers you to make data-driven decisions that enhance your well-being. For example, if you consistently notice digestive discomfort during a specific phase, you might experiment with dietary adjustments. Or, if your creativity surges in the follicular phase, you could align your work on creative projects to this period for maximum efficacy.

Regularly review your tracking data – a monthly check-in is a good practice. Assess what's working and what isn't. Celebrate the successes, no matter how small, and consider what adjustments could be made to address any challenges. This is not a one-time evaluation but a continuous process that echoes the cyclical nature of your body.

Lastly, be patient with yourself. Cycle alignment is a personal journey, and it may take several cycles to fully understand and harmonize with your body's rhythms. Each cycle is an opportunity to learn more about yourself and to refine your approach. Trust in the process, and allow your personal cycle syncing plan to be a living document that grows and changes as you do.

By embracing a systematic and data-driven approach to tracking your progress, you are equipping yourself with the knowledge and flexibility needed to create a cycle-syncing plan that genuinely resonates with your body's innate wisdom. This is not just a plan but a pathway to a more attuned and empowered you.

Chapter Summary

- Begin by tracking your menstrual cycle phases: menstrual, follicular, ovulatory, and luteal, noting symptoms and emotional and physical states in each phase.
- Assess how your current lifestyle, including activities, work, social life, and exercise, aligns with your cycle phases.
- Evaluate your nutrition, ensuring you consume phase-appropriate foods that support your hormonal fluctuations.
- Monitor sleep patterns and their correlation with your cycle, as hormonal shifts can affect sleep quality.
- Reflect on stress levels and management techniques, considering the impact of stress on hormonal balance.
- Set specific, measurable goals and intentions for cycle synchronization, aligned with personal values and aspirations.
- Design a personalized cycle alignment strategy, adjusting activities, diet, and tasks to each cycle phase.
- Implement and adjust your plan based on body responses, maintaining flexibility and a non-judgmental attitude towards yourself.

10

THE FUTURE OF CYCLE ALIGNMENT

As we delve into the realm of cycle alignment, it is essential to recognize that this field is not static but dynamic and burgeoning with potential. The concept of cycle alignment has gained traction in recent years. However, the future holds even more promise as emerging research and developments unfold, offering deeper insights and more refined approaches to this personalized health strategy.

One of the most exciting areas of development is the increasing understanding of the molecular and physiological mechanisms behind the menstrual cycle. Scientists are beginning to unravel the complex interplay of hormones, such as estrogen and progesterone, and their systemic effects on the body. This research not only reveals why specific symptoms manifest during different phases of the cycle but also how we might mitigate them effectively. For example, studies are exploring how fluctuations in hormone levels influence mood, energy, metabolism, and even the microbiome, which could lead to more nuanced cycle-syncing protocols.

Another promising avenue of research is investigating the impact of cycle syncing on various health conditions. Preliminary studies suggest that aligning lifestyle choices with hormonal fluctuations could potentially alleviate symptoms of conditions like polycystic ovary syndrome, endometriosis, and premenstrual syndrom. As research progresses, cycle synchronization could become a cornerstone of treatment plans for these and other hormone-related disorders.

The potential of cycle synchronization extends beyond symptom management. There is a growing body of evidence to suggest that it could play a role in enhancing overall well-being and performance. For example, by syncing exercise routines with the menstrual cycle, women may optimize their workouts, improve recovery, and even prevent injuries. Similarly, aligning nutrition with hormonal changes could maximize nutrient absorption and support metabolic health.

The implications of these developments are vast. As we gain a more sophisticated understanding of the menstrual cycle's influence on the body, cycle alignment could evolve into a highly personalized form of health optimization. It could empower individuals to manage symptoms and enhance their physical and mental performance, tailor their nutrition, and even improve their long-term health outcomes.

In the future, we may see the development of comprehensive cycle alignment programs that are as commonplace as general dietary and fitness plans are today. These programs would be backed by robust scientific research and could be tailored to each individual's unique hormonal profile, lifestyle, and health goals.

As we stand on the cusp of these advancements, it is clear that the future of cycle synchronization is bright. With continued research and development, this approach has the potential to transform the way women live in harmony with their bodies, unlocking a new paradigm of personalized health and wellness.

The Role of Technology in Cycle Alignment

As we delve into the transformative potential of technology in cycle alignment, it is essential to recognize its profound impact on personal health management. The advent of sophisticated apps and wearable devices has revolutionized the way individuals can monitor and understand their menstrual cycles, offering a personalized approach to health that was once unattainable.

Integrating technology into cycle alignment is not merely a matter of convenience but a profound expansion of personal agency and self-knowledge. Women and individuals with menstrual cycles are now equipped with tools that provide insights into their hormonal fluctuations, fertility windows, and potential health issues. These technological advancements can demystify the menstrual cycle, transforming it from a taboo subject into a wellspring of valuable health data.

Wearable technology, in particular, has taken the forefront in this revolution. Devices that track physiological parameters such as body temperature, heart rate, and sleep patterns are becoming increasingly sophisticated. They offer real-time data that can help predict energy levels, mood changes, and nutritional needs when correlated with menstrual cycle phases. This level of detail empowers individuals to make informed decisions about exercise, diet, social engagements, and work productivity, all tailored to the rhythm of their cycles.

Moreover, the data collected by these technologies is not only beneficial on an individual level but also has the potential to contribute to a larger pool of research. With user consent, anonymized health data can be invaluable for scientific studies, leading to a deeper understanding of menstrual health and its connection to overall well-being. This collective knowledge could drive the development of more effective treatments for menstrual-related disorders and pave the way for a future where cycle alignment is not an alternative method but a standard practice in personalized healthcare.

The role of artificial intelligence (AI) in this domain cannot be overstated. AI algorithms are becoming increasingly adept at pattern recognition, learning from the menstrual cycle data input by users to provide more accurate predictions and personalized health insights. This could lead to AI-powered virtual health assistants that track and analyze cycle data and offer recommendations for optimizing physical and mental health based on an individual's unique cycle patterns.

However, with the rise of technology comes the imperative responsibility to address privacy concerns. The intimate nature of menstrual health data necessitates stringent security measures to protect user information. Developers and companies behind cycle alignment technologies must prioritize data encryption and ethical data usage policies to maintain trust and ensure that users' personal health information is safeguarded against unauthorized access.

In conclusion, the role of technology in cycle alignment is a testament to the remarkable strides made in personal health management. By harnessing the power of wearable devices, apps, and AI, individuals gain unprecedented control over their health and well-being. As we continue to explore these technologies' capabilities, we must advocate for responsible data practices and continue to educate on the importance of menstrual health, ensuring that the future of cycle alignment is not only technologically advanced but also inclusive, secure, and empowering.

Expanding the Conversation: Education and Advocacy

In pursuing a future where cycle alignment is not only a well-understood concept but also a widely accepted practice, the expansion of conversation through education and advocacy is a pivotal step. This expansion is not merely about spreading awareness; it is about embedding the knowledge of menstrual health and cycle alignment into the fabric of society, thereby empowering individuals to make informed decisions about their bodies and overall well-being.

Education, in this context, takes on a multi-faceted approach. It begins in the classroom, where comprehensive sex education should include detailed information on menstrual cycles and the impact they have on an individual's physical and emotional state. By introducing cycle alignment as a topic of study, educators can provide young people with the tools to understand and work with their bodies rather than against them. When imparted early, this knowledge can lay the groundwork for a lifetime of informed health choices and self-awareness.

Beyond the classroom, education must also permeate into the healthcare system. From general practitioners to specialists, medical professionals should be equipped with the latest research and understanding of cycle alignment. This ensures that when patients come with questions or seek advice on menstrual health, they receive guidance that is not only empathetic but also scientifically sound and tailored to their unique rhythms.

Advocacy is crucial in normalizing the conversation around menstrual health and cycle syncing. Advocates can work to dismantle the taboos and stigmas that have long shrouded discussions of menstruation. Advocates can foster a culture of openness and acceptance by creating platforms where individuals feel safe and supported in sharing their experiences. This, in turn, can influence policy-making, leading to menstrual health considerations in the workplace, such as flexible scheduling and environments that accommodate the varying phases of the menstrual cycle.

Moreover, advocacy efforts can help to secure funding for further research into cycle alignment. With a robust body of evidence, the potential benefits of cycle syncing can be more widely recognized, leading to its integration into health and wellness programs. This could pave the way for apps and technology, discussed in the previous section, to be more than just personal tools; they could become part of a more significant, systemic approach to health management.

Expanding the conversation through education and advocacy is about creating a world where cycle syncing is not an esoteric concept but a common practice. It is about ensuring that everyone has the knowledge and support to harness the power of their menstrual cycle, leading to a future where cycle alignment is as routine as any other aspect of health and wellness.

Building a Community Around Menstrual Health

In the pursuit of a future where cycle synchronization is not only understood but also embraced, the creation of a robust community around menstrual health stands as a pivotal step. This community, envisioned as a collective of individuals from diverse backgrounds, would serve as a sanctuary for sharing experiences, offering support, and disseminating knowledge about the intricacies of menstrual cycles and the broader implications of hormonal health.

The foundation of such a community is rooted in the recognition that menstrual health is not a niche concern but a universal aspect of human biology that affects half of the population directly and the other half indirectly. By fostering open dialogue and creating safe spaces, both virtual and physical, individuals can learn from one another, share their triumphs and challenges, and normalize the conversation around menstruation and cycle alignment.

To build this community, a multi-faceted approach is necessary. Firstly, leveraging technology to connect individuals across geographical boundaries can provide a platform for those seeking guidance and camaraderie. Online forums, social media groups, and dedicated apps can offer resources and facilitate discussions that empower individuals to take charge of their menstrual health through cycle alignment.

Secondly, local meet-ups and workshops can complement online interactions, providing a tangible sense of community. These gatherings can range from educational seminars led by healthcare professionals to informal support groups. By meeting face-to-face, individuals can form stronger bonds and a sense of belonging, essential for sustaining engagement and fostering a supportive network.

Furthermore, collaboration with healthcare providers is crucial. By involving experts in the field, the community can ensure that the information shared is accurate and up-to-date. Healthcare professionals can also benefit from such a community by gaining insights into the real-world experiences of those they treat, leading to more empathetic and personalized care.

In addition to these efforts, the community must be inclusive and acknowledge the diversity of experiences with menstrual health. Recognizing that menstrual cycles and hormonal changes affect everyone differently, the community should celebrate this diversity and strive to cater to various needs and perspectives. This inclusivity extends to individuals with various health conditions, gender identities, and cultural backgrounds, all of whom should find their place within the community.

Lastly, the community should not only be a source of support but also a force for change. By uniting individuals who are informed and passionate about menstrual health, the community can advocate for better resources, research, and recognition of the importance of cycle syncing in public health agendas.

In essence, building a community around menstrual health is about creating a movement that champions the well-being of individuals through shared knowledge, mutual support, and collective action. Through this community, the future of cycle alignment can be realized, ensuring that every individual can live in harmony with their body's natural rhythms.

Envisioning a Society in Sync with Cycles

In the tapestry of human health and well-being, menstrual health has often been a thread that's been overlooked or hidden away. However, as we look to the future, we can envision a society that not only acknowledges but also embraces the concept of cycle alignment. This is a future where the natural rhythms of the menstrual cycle are harmoniously integrated into the fabric of daily life, fostering an environment that supports the physical, emotional, and mental health of those who menstruate.

Imagine a world where workplaces, educational institutions, and social settings are all tuned to the menstrual cycle. In this society, the stigma surrounding menstruation dissipates, replaced by a culture of openness and understanding. Work schedules and academic deadlines could be more flexible, accommodating the varying energy levels and cognitive states associated with the different phases of the menstrual cycle. This would not only enhance productivity but also promote a sense of well-being and respect for the body's natural processes.

In such a society, menstrual health education is comprehensive and begins early. Both young people and adults are equipped with the knowledge to understand and work with their cycles rather than against them. This education extends beyond biological aspects, encompassing the emotional and psychological influences of hormonal fluctuations. With this knowledge, individuals can make informed decisions about diet, exercise, social engagements, and work tasks that align with their cycle phases.

Healthcare systems in this envisioned future are more responsive and personalized. Medical professionals are trained in cycle alignment, enabling them to provide care tailored to the individual's cycle phase. This could lead to more effective treatments for menstrual-related disorders and a greater emphasis on preventative care. Technology, too, plays a pivotal role, with apps and devices designed to track and analyze menstrual cycles, offering insights and recommendations for optimal living in accordance with one's cycle.

In the realm of personal relationships, cycle alignment fosters empathy and communication. Partners and family members are more attuned to the needs and experiences of those who menstruate, leading to stronger, more supportive bonds. Social plans can be made with consideration of one's cycle, ensuring that activities are aligned with the energy and mood of the individual.

Furthermore, the future of cycle alignment extends to public policy. Governments and institutions could implement policies supporting menstrual health, such as providing menstrual products in public restrooms and ensuring access to health education and care. These policies would not only support those who menstruate but also signal a broader commitment to public health and gender equality.

In this future, cycle alignment is not a niche concept but a widespread practice that enhances the quality of life. It is a testament to a society that values the health and well-being of all its members, recognizing the profound impact that syncing with natural cycles can have on individual and collective prosperity.

As we move forward, the potential of cycle alignment is boundless. It offers a pathway to a more attuned, empathetic, and health-conscious society. By embracing the natural rhythms of the menstrual cycle, we can create a future that is not only in sync with our bodies but also with our potential for growth and harmony.

Chapter Summary

- The future of cycle synchronization is promising, with ongoing research into how diet, exercise, and lifestyle can be tailored to the menstrual cycle phases.
- Scientists are uncovering how hormonal fluctuations affect mood, energy, metabolism, and the microbiome, which may lead to more effective cycle alignment methods.
- Preliminary studies indicate that cycle syncing could help alleviate symptoms of hormonal disorders like PCOS, endometriosis, and PMS.
- Cycle alignment may enhance overall well-being and performance, optimizing workouts, recovery, and nutrient absorption based on menstrual cycle phases.
- Technology, including apps and wearable devices, is revolutionizing cycle alignment by providing personalized menstrual cycle data and health insights.
- Artificial intelligence could further personalize health recommendations based on menstrual cycle patterns, but privacy and data security are paramount concerns.
- Education and advocacy are key to normalizing cycle alignment, with a need for comprehensive menstrual health education and informed healthcare professionals.
- Building a community around menstrual health can offer support, share knowledge, and advocate for public health policies that recognize the importance and benefits of cycle alignment.

YOUR JOURNEY BEYOND THE PAGES

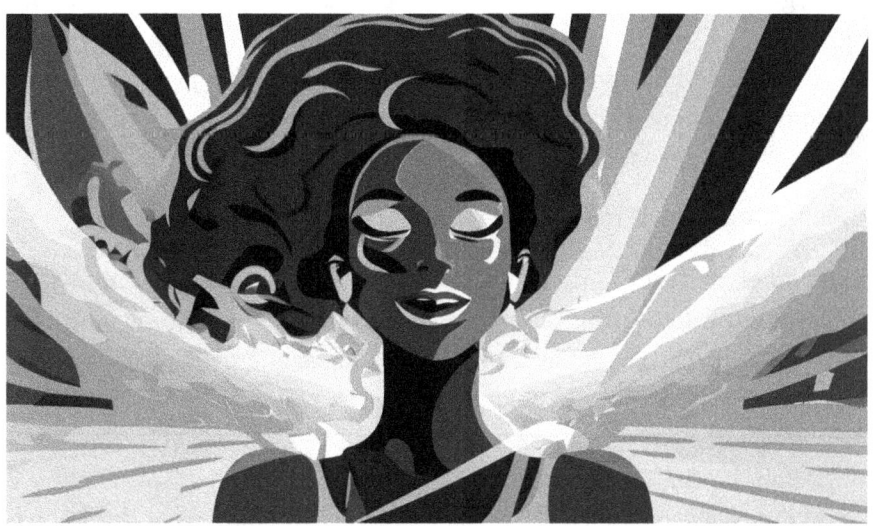

As we reach the concluding chapter of this book, it's time to pause and reflect on what you've learned and how far you've come. Think back to the beginning of this book and consider the changes in how you now understand and relate to your cycle. This reflection is crucial in solidifying the knowledge and practices you've acquired.

Take a moment to appreciate the growth in your self-awareness and the proactive steps you've taken to align your daily life with your cycle's rhythm. Whether you've made dietary adjustments, modified your exercise routine, or found new ways to manage stress, each change contributes to a healthier, more balanced you.

Use journaling or quiet contemplation to process your journey. Consider which chapters resonated the most and why. Reflect on how your perspective on your cycle has shifted and what this means for your future.

Acknowledging your journey is also about recognizing that learning and growth are ongoing processes. There may have been challenges along the way, but each one has offered valuable lessons and opportunities for personal development.

As you close this book, remember that the end of this reading is just the beginning of a lifelong practice. Keep revisiting these pages and your reflections as you evolve and deepen your connection with your cycle. Your journey with your body's natural rhythms doesn't stop here—it's a continuous path of discovery and empowerment.

Celebrating Your Wins

Remember to take a moment every now and then to celebrate your achievements. Recognize the progress you've made in aligning your lifestyle with your cycle. Whether it's feeling more energized, experiencing less discomfort, or finding greater balance in your life, these are significant milestones worth acknowledging.

Celebrate the small victories as well as the big ones. You may have started to notice patterns in your energy levels and have used this knowledge to plan your activities more effectively. Or perhaps you've found that certain foods help you feel better at different times of the month. No matter how minor they seem, these insights and changes are steps towards a more harmonious life.

Sharing your successes can be incredibly powerful. It not only reinforces your achievements but also encourages others to explore their paths to cycle alignment. Whether you share with friends, family, or a wider audience, your story can inspire and guide.

Creating a personal ritual to celebrate these wins can also be beneficial. It could be as simple as taking a moment at the end of each cycle to reflect on what went well or treating yourself to something special as a reward for your efforts. This act of celebration helps to solidify the positive changes you've made.

Remember, regardless of size, each win is a step forward in your journey. These accomplishments are the results and motivators that propel you toward continued growth and well-being. So, take the time to honor your hard work and the positive outcomes that have come from it. Your journey doesn't end here; each cycle brings new opportunities to build on these successes and continue to thrive.

Overcoming Challenges

As we draw the final threads of our narrative together, it's essential to acknowledge that aligning with your cycle is not without its hurdles. You may have encountered obstacles along the way, or perhaps you're still navigating through them. It's essential to recognize that these challenges are a natural part of the journey, and overcoming them is a testament to your resilience.

Remember, the road to harmony with your cycle is much like the cycle itself—dynamic and ever-changing. There will be days when everything falls into place effortlessly and others when it feels like an uphill climb. During these times, your strength and determination are truly tested, and it's also when the most profound growth can occur.

If you've faced setbacks, take a moment to reflect on what they've taught you. Each challenge is an opportunity to learn more about your body and yourself. They prompt you to adapt, to seek out new strategies, and to reach out for support when needed. Embrace these lessons, for they are valuable guides on your path forward.

Lean on the community of fellow cycle explorers you've met along the way, whether in person or through the vast connections of the online world. There is strength in numbers, and the shared wisdom of others can provide comfort and practical advice as you continue to navigate your journey.

As you move beyond this book, carry with you the understanding that challenges are not roadblocks but stepping stones to greater self-awareness and empowerment. With each obstacle you overcome, you pave the way for a smoother journey ahead for yourself and others who walk the path beside you.

So, as we close this chapter, remember that the true essence of overcoming is not in never facing difficulties but rising each time we fall. Your journey with your cycle is a continuous evolution, where each challenge surmounted adds a new layer of strength to your story. Keep this spirit of perseverance close to your heart, and step forward with confidence, knowing that you are equipped to meet and master whatever lies ahead.

Continuing the Cycle Alignment Journey

As we approach the end of this written voyage, remember that the true journey doesn't have a final destination. The practice of aligning with your cycle is an ongoing adventure that continues to unfold each month. It's a lifelong commitment to listening to your body and responding to its needs with care and understanding.

Maintaining the harmony between your lifestyle and your cycle requires consistent attention and nurturing. It's like tending to a garden; regular care ensures it flourishes. Keep the principles you've learned in this book close to your heart, and integrate them into the fabric of your daily life. Let them become as natural to you as breathing.

Staying motivated can be challenging, but remember why you started this journey. Revisit your reflections and celebrate your wins to remind yourself of the positive changes you've experienced. This is the fuel that will keep your inner fire burning brightly.

As you move forward, continue to explore and deepen your understanding of your body. Stay curious and open to new research, insights, and strategies that can enhance your cycle alignment practice. Knowledge is a powerful tool, and there's always more to learn.

Encourage yourself to be flexible and adaptable. As your life changes, so may your cycle and how you align with it. Embrace these changes as part of life's natural ebb and flow, and adjust your practices accordingly.

Remember, this book is a starting point, a foundation upon which you can build a more prosperous, more attuned relationship with your cycle. Keep it as a trusted guide, but also trust in your wisdom and the wisdom of your body. You have all the tools you need to continue this journey with confidence and grace.

So, as we part ways in text, know that your cycle alignment journey is just beginning. Carry forward the lessons, the love, and the commitment to your well-being that you've cultivated here. Your path ahead is bright with the promise of continued growth, balance, and empowerment.

Looking Forward

Now, let's cast our gaze forward to the horizon of your journey. The chapters behind us have been a map to guide you, but the path ahead is yours to forge with the wisdom and understanding you've gained. The future of aligning with your cycle is a canvas stretched out before you, ready for your continued exploration and growth.

Envision a world where the knowledge you now hold is shared and celebrated—a world where the cycles of our bodies are honored as a source of insight and strength. You are now a beacon in this movement, a pioneer in living in harmony with your body's natural rhythms. Embrace this role and consider how you can inspire others to embark on their journeys of discovery and alignment.

The conversation around menstrual health and cycle awareness is ever-evolving; you are part of that evolution. Advocate for this awareness in your circles and help to weave this understanding into the fabric of society. Each voice that joins this chorus amplifies the message, bringing us closer to a future where cycle alignment is not just a personal practice but a collective awakening.

As you close this book, remember that the end of this reading is just one milestone in your lifelong relationship with your cycle. Continue to nurture this relationship, listen, and respond to your body with love and respect. The empowerment you've found within these pages is a flame that will light your way through all the cycles to come.

So, dear reader, as you step beyond the pages of this book, carry with you the courage, the knowledge, and the joy you've discovered. Let them be your companions as you journey forward, creating a life that is not only in sync with your cycle but also in tune with the deepest parts of yourself.

Here's to the future—a future where each of us lives in full bloom, aligned with the powerful rhythms of our bodies, and where every cycle is a celebration of our innate wisdom and beauty.

WOMAN'S HORMONE HANDBOOK

UNLOCK THE SECRETS OF FEMALE
HORMONAL HEALTH FOR LIFELONG
BALANCE AND VITALITY

EMBRACING HORMONAL HARMONY

Welcome to the intricate world of hormones, the unsung heroes orchestrating the vast symphony of womanhood. These potent chemical messengers are pivotal in every chapter of a woman's life, from the awakening of puberty to the transformative waves of menopause.

Every day and night, your hormones work harmoniously to create the rich and dynamic experience of being a woman. Hormones like estrogen and progesterone ebb and flow, shaping reproductive health and influencing everything from your mood to your metabolism.

The "Woman's Hormone Handbook" is designed to illuminate these complex interactions, providing you with the knowledge to understand your body's signals and act upon them. In this book, we'll embark on an enlightening journey to decode the whispers and roars of your hormonal landscape. Understanding these signals is crucial, as they influence not just physical health but also emotional well-being and mental clarity. As we unfold the pages of this guide, you'll gain insights into how to harmonize your body's natural rhythms, empowering you to live with vitality and grace.

You'll discover how to listen to your body's hormonal cues and respond with informed, nurturing choices. Whether navigating the tides of fertility or seeking solace in the flux of hormonal shifts, this book is your compass to a balanced and vibrant existence. It is more than a guide; it celebrates the female body's innate wisdom. Together, we'll explore the beauty and challenges of each hormonal shift, equipping you with the tools to thrive through every phase of life.

The Endocrine System

Imagine the endocrine system as a magnificent orchestra, with each gland playing a vital role in the symphony of your body's functions. This complex network of glands and hormones works in unison to regulate everything from growth and metabolism to mood and reproduction. We'll delve into the intricacies of this system, demystifying how it conducts the rhythms of daily life, and you'll learn how each gland and hormone can affect your well-being. Disruptions in this delicate balance may lead to conditions such as thyroid disorders or adrenal fatigue, which can profoundly impact your quality of life.

Understanding the endocrine system's melody is essential to mastering your hormonal health. With the knowledge you'll gain from these pages, you'll be equipped to fine-tune your body's hormonal orchestra, ensuring that each gland plays its part beautifully and you experience the full, rich symphony of optimal health.

Hormonal Challenges and Triumphs

Navigating the ebb and flow of hormones is a central part of life. In this book, we'll also explore the common hormonal challenges many women encounter, acknowledging the struggles and celebrating the triumphs that come with each. Conditions like Polycystic Ovary Syndrome and thyroid imbalances are more than mere inconveniences; they are puzzles that, when solved, can unlock a new level of wellness and self-understanding.

You'll find empowering strategies to manage and mitigate their effects, turning a challenge into a victory for your health. We'll explore how to confidently navigate their symptoms, using both time-tested remedies and modern medical advancements.

A Holistic Approach to Hormone Health

This book doesn't shy away from the role of medical interventions, including hormone replacement therapy and supplements. Instead, it places these within a larger context of self-care and informed choice. Hormonal health is not merely the absence of disease; it's a state of complete harmony where lifestyle, nutrition, and medical care converge. By embracing a holistic approach, you'll learn to navigate the nuances of your hormonal health, crafting a personalized plan that resonates with your body's needs and your life's unique demands.

Your Companion on the Journey to Well-being

The "Woman's Hormone Handbook" is your guide to a more vibrant, balanced you. It is more than a mere collection of facts and advice; it is a steadfast companion on your personal journey to well-being. As you turn each page, you'll find a supportive guide that understands the intricacies of your body's hormonal ebb and flow. This book is a testament to the belief that knowledge is power—the power to heal, balance, and thrive.

Embarking on this journey, you'll be equipped with a deep understanding of how hormones impact every facet of your health. From the physical changes of puberty to the emotional swings of menopause, this handbook provides clarity and comfort. It's a resource you can return to time and again, finding answers to your questions and solace in shared experiences.

The journey to hormonal well-being is not a straight path—it's a winding road filled with discoveries and learning opportunities. As your companion, this book offers easy to understand explanations and practical, real-world applications. It empowers you to make informed decisions about your health, whether you're considering dietary changes, lifestyle adjustments, or medical treatments.

Above all, this book celebrates womanhood in all its complexity. It encourages you to embrace your body's signals, listen intently, and respond with love and care. Your journey to hormonal harmony is a profound one, and with this book in hand, you're never alone. Together, we'll navigate the path to a balanced and fulfilling life where well-being is your destination. So, are you ready to begin?

1
UNDERSTANDING HORMONES: THE BASICS

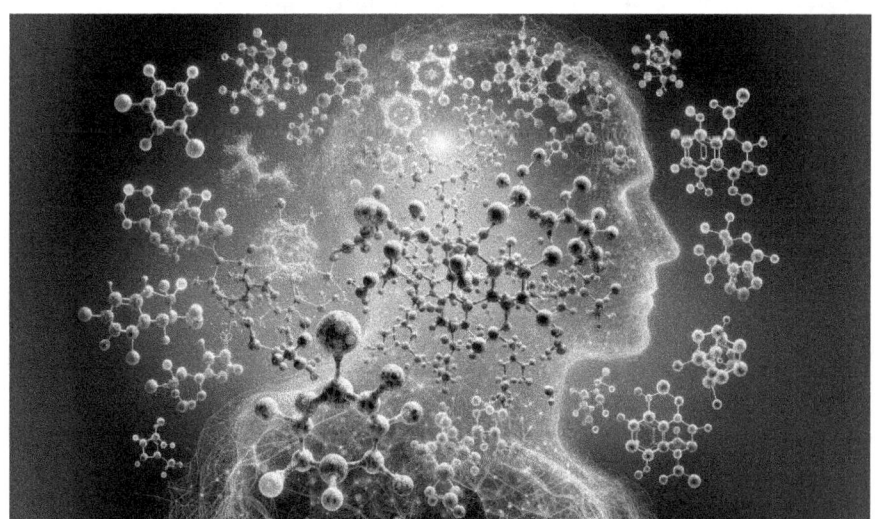

I magine your body as a complex network, a bustling city where communication is vital to maintaining order and balance. In this city, hormones are the messengers, the whispers and shouts that travel through the bloodstream, carrying vital information from one part of the body to another. They are the chemical signals that orchestrate many bodily functions, from growth and metabolism to mood and reproduction.

Hormones are produced by various glands and organs within the body, each with a specific set of responsibilities. These glands are like unique broadcasting stations, sending messages to target cells equipped with the right receivers – hormone receptors. When a hormone docks onto its receptor, it delivers its message, prompting the cell to perform a particular action or initiate a series of events.

The beauty of hormones lies in their diversity and specificity. Some, like insulin, regulate the sugar level in our blood, ensuring that our cells receive the energy they need. Others, such as estrogen and progesterone, play pivotal roles in the reproductive system, influencing menstrual cycles, pregnancy, and even the health of our bones and heart.

But hormones are not solo artists; they perform in a finely-tuned ensemble. The balance between different hormones is crucial. Too much or too little of a single hormone can disrupt this balance, leading to a variety of health issues. For women, this balance is particularly delicate, as their bodies undergo significant hormonal changes throughout life – from the onset of puberty to the transition of menopause.

Understanding hormones is akin to learning a new language, one that can explain why we feel the way we do, why our bodies change over time, and how we can better support our health by listening to the subtle yet powerful signals they send us. As we delve deeper into the world of hormones, we'll discover how this intricate system of chemical messengers influences our physical well-being, emotions, and behaviors.

So, let's continue our journey into the next section, where we'll explore the endocrine system – the network of glands that compose the grand symphony of hormone production and regulation in our bodies. By understanding this system, we'll gain insights into how to maintain harmony within, ensuring that each gland plays its part beautifully in the concert of our health.

The Endocrine System: A Symphony of Glands

Imagine an orchestra, each musician poised with an instrument, ready to play their part in a complex musical piece. This is akin to the endocrine system in our bodies—a collection of glands that work in concert to produce and release hormones, the body's chemical messengers. Each gland in the endocrine system has a specific role, much like each musician in an orchestra has a particular part to play. Together, they create a harmony that regulates various bodily functions, from growth and metabolism to reproduction and mood.

The maestro of this symphony is the hypothalamus, a small but mighty region of the brain. It's the conductor, directing the pituitary gland, often called the 'master gland,' through signals that determine the release of hormones. The pituitary gland, in response, sends its own signals to other glands in the body, such as the thyroid, adrenals, and the reproductive organs—the ovaries in women.

The thyroid gland, nestled in the front of your neck, plays the notes that regulate your metabolism, energy levels, and even how warm you feel. It's like the orchestra's string section, setting the pace and tone for many bodily functions.

The adrenal glands, perched atop your kidneys like tiny hats, produce hormones like cortisol and adrenaline. These are the brass instruments that sound the alarm and energize the body in times of stress or excitement.

For women, the ovaries are the soloists of the hormone symphony, producing estrogen and progesterone. These hormones are central to reproductive health, influencing menstrual cycles, pregnancy, and even the transition into menopause.

Each gland works in response to the others, with feedback loops fine-tuning the performance. Suppose one musician plays too loudly or softly or misses a cue. In that case, the harmony is disrupted, leading to various health issues. For example, an overactive thyroid can cause symptoms like anxiety and weight loss. In contrast, an underactive thyroid might lead to fatigue and weight gain.

Maintaining this delicate balance is crucial for overall health, and it's especially important for women, whose hormonal needs change throughout their lives. Understanding how these glands work together helps us appreciate the complexity and beauty of our bodies. It underscores the importance of taking care of our hormonal health.

As we move forward, we'll explore the unique relationship women have with their hormones and how this connection influences their health at every stage of life. Just as every note in a symphony is essential to the beauty of the whole piece, every hormone in your body plays a vital role in your overall well-being.

Hormones and Women: A Unique Relationship

In the intricate dance of the endocrine system, women's bodies play a particularly complex tune. Hormones, those chemical messengers that traverse our bloodstream to regulate physiology and behavior, profoundly impact women's health. Their influence begins at puberty and wends its way through the phases of adulthood, from the potential for pregnancy to the transition of menopause.

For women, hormones do more than just regulate the reproductive system. They are pivotal in determining many bodily functions, including but not limited to metabolism, bone density, and even mood. Estrogen and progesterone, the primary female sex hormones, are often the stars of the show. They're supported by a cast of others like testosterone, which women produce in smaller amounts, and thyroid hormones, cortisol, and insulin.

The relationship between women and their hormones is unique, not only because of the cyclical nature of the female reproductive system but also because of how these hormones interact with each other and different body systems. For instance, estrogen plays a crucial role in maintaining healthy bones, and a drop in its levels during menopause can lead to an increased risk of osteoporosis. Similarly, hormonal fluctuations can affect mental health, with some women experiencing mood swings, anxiety, or depression as hormone levels ebb and flow during the menstrual cycle, pregnancy, or menopause.

Understanding this relationship is crucial because it underscores the importance of hormone balance in overall health. When hormones are in harmony, they facilitate the smooth operation of bodily functions. However, when imbalances occur, they can lead to a range of health issues, from menstrual irregularities and skin problems to more serious conditions like polycystic ovary syndrome (PCOS) or thyroid disorders.

Moreover, the influence of hormones extends beyond physical health. They can affect emotional well-being, influencing how you feel and perceive the world around you. It's not uncommon for women to notice changes in their emotional state at different points in their menstrual cycle, and these shifts are a testament to the powerful effects hormones have on the brain and nervous system.

It's also important to recognize that everyone's hormonal journey is unique. Factors such as genetics, lifestyle, stress levels, and environmental exposures can all influence hormone health. This means that while there are general patterns and shared experiences, each woman's hormonal profile and how it affects her health and well-being is highly individual.

By embracing a holistic view of hormone health, you can better understand your body and take proactive steps toward maintaining hormonal balance. This might include lifestyle changes such as diet and exercise, stress management techniques, or, when necessary, seeking medical advice and treatment options.

In the next part of our exploration, we will delve into the lifecycle of female hormones, tracing their ebbs and flows from the onset of menstruation to menopause. This journey will illuminate not only the biological milestones of a woman's life but also how these hormonal shifts can be navigated to maintain health and vitality at every stage.

The Lifecycle of Female Hormones

As we delve into the intricate world of female hormones, we must recognize that their journey is not static. The lifecycle of female hormones is a dynamic and continuous process, evolving from puberty through menopause. This journey is marked by a symphony of hormonal fluctuations that influence reproductive health and play a significant role in overall well-being.

Let's begin with puberty, a time of significant change as the body transitions from childhood into reproductive maturity. This period is characterized by the activation of the hypothalamic-pituitary-gonadal axis, which orchestrates the production and regulation of critical hormones like estrogen and progesterone. These hormones are responsible for the development of secondary sexual characteristics and the initiation of menstrual cycles.

As a young woman's body adapts to these changes, the menstrual cycle becomes a central aspect of hormonal health. Each cycle can be divided into distinct phases: the follicular phase, ovulation, and the luteal phase. During the follicular phase, the hormone estrogen rises, leading to the maturation of an ovarian follicle. Ovulation then marks the release of an egg. This moment hinges on a delicate balance of luteinizing hormone (LH) and follicle-stimulating hormone (FSH). Following ovulation, the luteal phase increases progesterone, preparing the uterine lining for potential pregnancy.

If pregnancy does not occur, the cycle concludes with menstruation, and the hormonal dance begins anew. It's important to acknowledge that while this cycle is described in a neat sequence, many women experience variations in cycle length and hormone levels, which are entirely normal.

As women age, they eventually encounter perimenopause, the transitional period leading up to menopause. This stage can last several years and is marked by more pronounced hormonal fluctuations. Estrogen and progesterone levels may rise and fall unpredictably, leading to changes in menstrual patterns and, often, the onset of symptoms such as hot flashes, night sweats, and mood swings.

Finally, menopause is reached when a woman has not menstruated for 12 consecutive months. At this point, the ovaries have ceased releasing eggs and producing most of their estrogen. While menopause is a natural biological process, the decline in estrogen can have widespread effects on the body, including changes in bone density, cardiovascular health, and skin elasticity.

Throughout each of these stages, it's crucial to understand that hormone levels are not just reproductive signals; they influence a myriad of systems in the body. From emotional regulation to metabolic processes, hormones are integral to maintaining balance and health.

As we move forward, we will explore how disruptions in this delicate hormonal balance can lead to various disorders. By understanding the typical lifecycle of female hormones, we can better recognize when something may be amiss and take steps to address these issues with compassion and knowledge.

Common Hormonal Disorders in Women

As we delve deeper into the intricacies of hormone health, it's essential to understand that the delicate balance of hormones can sometimes be disrupted, leading to various disorders that can significantly impact a woman's quality of life. These disorders can manifest at any stage, from the onset of puberty to post-menopause, and understanding them is the first step towards managing and treating them effectively.

One of the most common hormonal disorders affecting women is Polycystic Ovary Syndrome (PCOS). This condition is characterized by an imbalance of reproductive hormones, which can lead to a variety of symptoms, including irregular menstrual cycles, acne, excessive hair growth, and difficulties with fertility. Women with PCOS may also experience insulin resistance, which can increase the risk of developing type 2 diabetes.

Another disorder that is frequently encountered is thyroid dysfunction, which can come in the form of hypothyroidism or hyperthyroidism. The thyroid gland plays a crucial role in regulating metabolism, and any imbalance can lead to symptoms such as weight gain or loss, fatigue, changes in heart rate, and mood disturbances. Hypothyroidism, where the thyroid produces insufficient hormones, is more common and can be particularly challenging for women, as it can also affect menstrual regularity and fertility.

Menstrual disorders such as premenstrual syndrome (PMS) and premenstrual dysphoric disorder (PMDD) also have a hormonal basis. While PMS is relatively common, and its symptoms—such as bloating, mood swings, and breast tenderness—are familiar to many, PMDD is a more severe form that can be debilitating. PMDD can cause extreme mood shifts and has a profound impact on a woman's emotional and physical well-being.

During the transition to menopause, known as perimenopause, women may experience hormonal fluctuations that can lead to symptoms like hot flashes, night sweats, sleep disturbances, and mood swings. This period can last several years and is a natural part of aging. Still, for some women, the symptoms can be severe enough to disrupt daily life.

Endometriosis is another condition that, while not solely a hormonal disorder, is influenced by hormonal activity. This painful condition occurs when tissue similar to the lining of the uterus grows outside of it, leading to severe pain, irregular bleeding, and potential fertility issues. Hormones play a role in the growth of this tissue, and managing hormonal levels can be a crucial aspect of treatment.

Lastly, hormonal imbalances can also lead to conditions such as osteoporosis, particularly after menopause, when the protective effects of estrogen decline. This can result in a decrease in bone density, making bones more fragile and susceptible to fractures.

Hormones are powerful messengers in our bodies. When their messages go awry, the effects can be far-reaching. However, many of these disorders can be treated effectively with proper diagnosis and management. It's essential to be attuned to your body and seek medical advice when you notice changes that could indicate a hormonal imbalance. By doing so, you can take proactive steps toward maintaining your hormonal health and overall well-being.

Chapter Summary

- Hormones are chemical messengers that regulate bodily functions, including growth, metabolism, mood, and reproduction. They are produced by various glands and organs.

- The balance of hormones is crucial for health, with imbalances causing issues; women's hormonal balance is particularly delicate due to life changes like puberty and menopause.
- The endocrine system consists of glands that produce hormones, with the hypothalamus and pituitary glands directing other glands like the thyroid and adrenals.
- Women have a unique relationship with hormones, affecting not just reproduction but also metabolism, bone density, and mood, with estrogen and progesterone playing central roles.
- Hormonal imbalances in women can lead to health issues like menstrual irregularities, PCOS, and thyroid disorders and also affect emotional well-being.
- The lifecycle of female hormones involves puberty, menstrual cycles, perimenopause, and menopause, impacting reproductive health and overall well-being.
- Common hormonal disorders in women include PCOS, thyroid dysfunction, menstrual disorders like PMS and PMDD, perimenopausal symptoms, endometriosis, and osteoporosis post-menopause.
- Understanding and managing hormonal health is crucial for women, with lifestyle changes and medical treatment helping to maintain balance and address disorders.

2
PUBERTY TO FERTILITY: THE REPRODUCTIVE YEARS

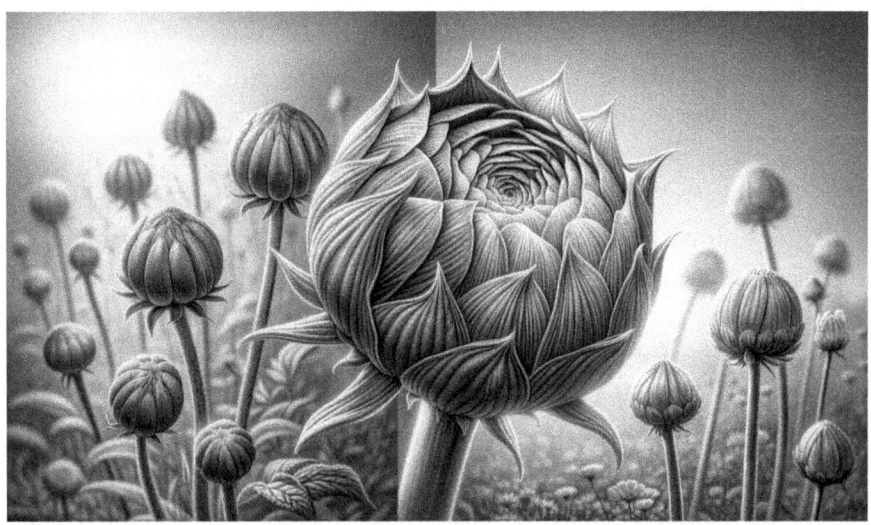

As the first whispers of womanhood begin, puberty ushers in a symphony of hormonal changes that transform the female body. This period of life is marked by the onset of menstruation, a milestone in reproductive maturity. It is the culmination of intricate hormonal events that deserve our understanding and respect.

The hormonal awakening typically begins between the ages of 8 and

13, when the hypothalamus, a master gland in the brain, releases gonadotropin-releasing hormone (GnRH). This hormone signals the pituitary gland to produce two other key players in the reproductive symphony: follicle-stimulating hormone (FSH) and luteinizing hormone (LH). These hormones travel through the bloodstream to the ovaries, which house thousands of dormant eggs.

In response to FSH and LH, the ovaries mature some of these eggs and produce the hormones estrogen and progesterone. Estrogen mainly plays a pivotal role in the development of secondary sexual characteristics, such as the growth of breasts, the widening of hips, and the appearance of pubic and underarm hair. It also contributes to the growth spurt that often accompanies puberty.

As estrogen levels rise, it triggers the thickening of the lining of the uterus, preparing it for the potential of pregnancy. If fertilization does not occur, the body must shed this lining, which leads to the first menstrual period, or menarche. The experience of menarche is as unique as the individual, with some girls greeting it with excitement, others with trepidation, and many with a mix of emotions.

It's important to note that the first few cycles can be irregular and may not even involve ovulation. This irregularity is expected as the body is still fine-tuning its hormonal communication. Over time, cycles generally settle into a more predictable pattern.

During this time, it is not uncommon for young women to experience a range of symptoms, from mood swings to cramps, as their bodies adjust to the ebb and flow of hormones. These experiences, while sometimes uncomfortable or confusing, are a normal part of the journey toward reproductive maturity.

As we embrace this hormonal awakening, providing support and education is crucial. Understanding the changes can empower young women to take charge of their health and well-being. Open conversations about menstruation, mood changes, and the physical transformations of puberty can demystify this natural process and foster a positive body image.

Remember, puberty is not just a biological event; it's a transition into a new phase of life with its own challenges and triumphs. As we move forward, we'll explore how the monthly rhythm of the menstrual cycle becomes a central part of a woman's life, influencing her health and well-being in profound ways.

The Menstrual Cycle: A Monthly Rhythm

As we journey through the reproductive years, the menstrual cycle is a testament to the intricate dance of hormones within a woman's body. This cycle, typically lasting around 28 days, though it can range from 21 to 35 days, is not just a biological process but a barometer of health and well-being.

At the heart of the menstrual cycle is the ebb and flow of hormones, primarily estrogen and progesterone, produced by the ovaries. These hormones work in a delicate balance, orchestrating the preparation of the uterus for potential pregnancy and the release of an egg during ovulation.

The cycle begins on the first day of menstruation, a phase commonly known as the period. This is when the lining of the uterus, which had thickened in preparation for a fertilized egg, is shed because pregnancy has not occurred. Menstruation can last anywhere from 2 to 7 days. While symptoms like cramping and mood swings can accompany it, it's a natural part of the cycle.

Following menstruation, the body enters the follicular phase. During this time, the pituitary gland releases follicle-stimulating hormone (FSH), which encourages the growth of ovarian follicles, each containing an immature egg. One of these follicles will become dominant and mature while the body reabsorbs the others.

As the dominant follicle grows, it produces more estrogen, which signals the lining of the uterus to thicken again, creating a nurturing environment for a potential embryo. This rise in estrogen also triggers a surge in luteinizing hormone (LH), which leads to the next pivotal event: ovulation.

Ovulation is the release of the mature egg from the ovary into the fallopian tube, where it awaits fertilization. This fertility window is narrow, with the egg remaining viable for about 24 hours. If sperm are present during this time, conception may occur.

Should fertilization not take place, the cycle progresses to the luteal phase. The ruptured follicle transforms into the corpus luteum, which secretes progesterone. Progesterone maintains the uterine lining, but without a pregnancy, its levels will eventually fall, leading to the shedding of the lining and the start of a new menstrual period.

Throughout these phases, women may experience a variety of symptoms, from the bloating and mood changes of premenstrual syndrome (PMS) to the heightened senses and energy around ovulation. It's important to remember that each woman's experience of her menstrual cycle is unique, and variations in cycle length, symptoms, and flow are all part of the spectrum of normal.

Understanding the menstrual cycle is more than just a matter of biology; it's about tuning into the rhythms of one's own body. By recognizing the patterns and signals of their cycles, women can gain insights into their overall health, plan for or prevent pregnancy, and make informed decisions about their reproductive health.

As we move forward, we'll delve deeper into the specifics of ovulation and fertility, unraveling the signs and processes crucial to conception and the continuation of these reproductive years.

Understanding Ovulation and Fertility

As we journey through the reproductive years, a fundamental aspect to grasp is the process of ovulation and its pivotal role in fertility. Ovulation is the release of an egg from one of the ovaries. This moment is both fleeting and fertile, marking a window of opportunity for conception.

Each month, in response to a symphony of hormonal signals, a select group of eggs, or oocytes, begin to mature within the ovarian follicles. Typically, one egg outpaces the others and reaches full maturity. This surge is orchestrated by a rise in follicle-stimulating hormone (FSH), which nudges the follicles into action, and luteinizing hormone (LH), which peaks just before ovulation, triggering the release of the egg.

The journey of the egg is a delicate voyage. Once released, it is swept into the fallopian tube, where it may meet sperm and become fertilized. This is where timing becomes crucial. The egg remains viable for about 12 to 24 hours post-ovulation, while sperm can survive in the female reproductive tract for up to five days. Therefore, the days leading up to and including ovulation constitute the fertile window.

Understanding one's fertility can be empowering. Many women learn to recognize the signs of ovulation, such as a change in cervical mucus, which becomes more transparent and more stretchy, akin to egg whites, and a slight rise in basal body temperature following ovulation. Others may experience ovulation pain, known as mittelschmerz, a dull ache, or a sharp twinge on one side of the lower abdomen.

Tracking these signs can be incredibly helpful for those trying to conceive, as it helps pinpoint the most fertile days. However, it's important to remember that each woman's cycle is unique, and these signs can vary widely. For some, ovulation can occur like clockwork, while for others, it may be more unpredictable.

For women not looking to conceive, understanding ovulation is equally essential. It informs choices around contraception and can shed light on various health conditions that may affect or be affected by the menstrual cycle. Moreover, it fosters a deeper connection with one's body, allowing for a proactive approach to reproductive health.

As we navigate the complexities of hormone health, it's clear that ovulation is not just a singular event but a cornerstone of the reproductive years. It's a dance of hormones, a convergence of timing, and a critical player in the journey from puberty to fertility. With this understanding, women can make informed decisions about their bodies, health, and futures.

Contraception and Hormonal Control

As we navigate the journey from puberty to fertility, it is equally important to discuss the choices available to women who wish to regulate their reproductive capabilities. Contraception and hormonal control are central to this discourse, offering women autonomy over their bodies and the freedom to decide if and when to have children.

Contraception comes in various forms, and hormonal methods are among the most popular and effective. These methods influence the natural hormonal rhythms that regulate ovulation and the menstrual cycle. Birth control pills, for instance, typically contain synthetic forms of estrogen and progesterone. By taking these hormones, a woman can prevent the release of an egg from her ovaries, thicken cervical mucus to block sperm, and thin the lining of the uterus to reduce the likelihood of implantation.

Another hormonal method includes the contraceptive patch, which releases hormones through the skin, and the vaginal ring, which releases hormones locally within the vagina. Both methods work similarly to the pill but offer convenience for those who prefer not to take a daily tablet.

Injectable contraceptives, such as the Depo-Provera shot, provide a longer-term solution, requiring administration every three months. The shot contains progestin, which suppresses ovulation and thickens cervical mucus.

For women seeking even longer-lasting contraception, hormonal implants and intrauterine devices (IUDs) can protect against pregnancy for several years. The implant, a tiny rod inserted under the skin of the arm, releases a steady dose of progestin. Hormonal IUDs, placed inside the uterus, release hormones locally to prevent fertilization.

While hormonal contraceptives are highly effective, they are not without potential side effects. Some women may experience changes in their menstrual cycle, mood swings, weight fluctuations, or other symptoms. It's essential to have an open dialogue with a healthcare provider to choose the most suitable method and to understand the possible effects on one's body and lifestyle.

Moreover, hormonal contraception can play a therapeutic role beyond birth control. For women with specific reproductive health issues, such as heavy menstrual bleeding, painful periods, or endometriosis, hormonal methods can offer significant relief. They regulate the menstrual cycle and can reduce the severity of symptoms, improving quality of life.

It is also important to acknowledge that while hormonal contraception can be empowering, it is not a one-size-fits-all solution. Each woman's body and hormonal balance are unique, and what works for one may not work for another. Personal preferences, health history, and future fertility plans are all critical factors in determining the best method of contraception.

In the next phase of our exploration into hormone health for women, we will delve into a condition that intimately ties into hormonal balance and reproductive health: Polycystic Ovary Syndrome (PCOS). This syndrome can affect a woman's hormonal levels, menstrual cycle, and overall health, and understanding its implications is vital for those who experience it.

Polycystic Ovary Syndrome: Insights and Management

In the journey of understanding hormone health for women, we've explored the nuances of contraception and hormonal control. Now we delve into a condition that intimately intertwines with these themes: Polycystic Ovary Syndrome, commonly known as PCOS. This syndrome is a complex endocrine disorder that affects an estimated one in ten women of reproductive age, making it a prevalent but often misunderstood condition.

PCOS is characterized by a combination of symptoms that can include irregular menstrual cycles, excess androgen levels (male hormones typically present in women in small amounts), and polycystic ovaries, which are enlarged and contain numerous small cysts. While the exact cause of PCOS remains unknown, it is believed to involve a combination of genetic and environmental factors, including insulin resistance and inflammation.

Women with PCOS often experience a range of symptoms that can vary in severity from mild to severe. These can include weight gain, acne, hirsutism (excessive hair growth on the face and body), thinning hair on the scalp, and difficulties with fertility. The emotional toll of managing these symptoms can be significant, leading to frustration and isolation.

Diagnosis of PCOS typically involves a review of medical history, physical examination, blood tests to measure hormone levels, and possibly an ultrasound to assess the ovaries. Because PCOS can mimic other health issues, it's crucial to rule out other potential causes of the symptoms.

Once diagnosed, management of PCOS is tailored to the individual's symptoms and concerns, such as managing irregular periods, acne, excess hair growth, and weight. Lifestyle changes, including diet and exercise, are pivotal in managing PCOS. A balanced diet rich in whole foods and low in processed carbohydrates can help manage insulin levels and support weight loss. Regular physical activity can also improve the body's sensitivity to insulin and aid in weight management.

For those struggling with fertility, medications that stimulate ovulation can be an option. Metformin, a medication commonly used to treat type 2 diabetes, has also been shown to improve insulin resistance in women with PCOS and can assist with ovulation.

Beyond physical symptoms, it's essential to address the psychological impact of PCOS. Support groups, counseling, and open dialogue with healthcare providers can provide invaluable emotional support. Women with PCOS may also face an increased risk for other health conditions, including type 2 diabetes, high blood pressure, and heart disease, making regular monitoring and preventive care essential.

In managing PCOS, the goal is not just to treat the symptoms but to empower women with the knowledge and resources they need to lead healthy, fulfilling lives. It's a journey that requires patience, understanding, and a compassionate approach to care. With the proper support and management strategies, women with PCOS can navigate the complexities of the condition and embrace their reproductive years with confidence and optimism.

Chapter Summary

- Puberty marks the beginning of a female's reproductive years, starting with hormonal changes and the onset of menstruation, typically between ages 8 and 13.

- The hypothalamus releases GnRH, which prompts the pituitary gland to produce FSH and LH, leading to egg maturation and hormone production in the ovaries.
- Estrogen is responsible for developing secondary sexual characteristics and preparing the uterus lining for potential pregnancy.
- The first menstrual cycles may be irregular and not involve ovulation, which is expected as the body adjusts its hormonal balance. Young women may experience mood swings, cramps, and other symptoms as they adjust to the hormonal changes during puberty. Open conversations and education about puberty can empower young women and promote a positive body image.
- The menstrual cycle, typically around 28 days, involves hormonal fluctuations that prepare the uterus for pregnancy and cause menstruation if no pregnancy occurs.
- Ovulation is the release of a mature egg, presenting a narrow window for fertilization; understanding this process is key for both conception and contraception.
- Hormonal contraceptives, like birth control pills, patches, rings, injections, implants, and IUDs, regulate ovulation and menstrual cycles, offering birth control and relief for specific reproductive health issues. Side effects of hormonal contraceptives can include menstrual changes and mood swings, and personal health history should guide contraceptive choices.
- Polycystic Ovary Syndrome (PCOS) affects one in ten women. It involves symptoms like irregular periods, excess androgens, and polycystic ovaries, with management tailored to individual needs.
- Lifestyle changes, medications for ovulation, and insulin resistance management are essential for PCOS treatment, along with support for the emotional impact of the condition.

3
PREGNANCY AND HORMONES: THE MIRACLE OF LIFE

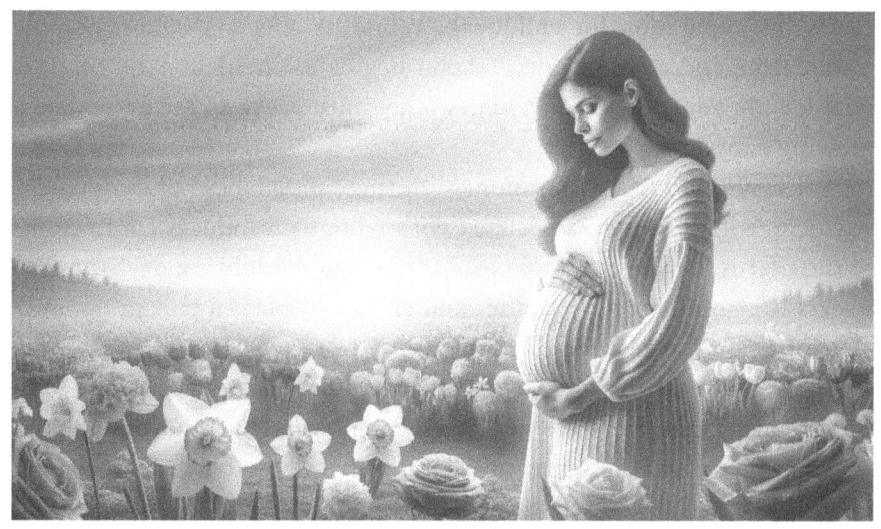

As we embark on this journey through the landscape of pregnancy, we'll begin to understand the profound hormonal shifts that occur within a woman's body. These changes are not just the backdrop to pregnancy; they are the very essence of it, orchestrating the development of new life with precision and care.

From the moment of conception, a woman's body becomes a finely tuned vessel for nurturing growth. The hormone human chorionic gonadotropin (hCG) is one of the first to enter the stage, signaling to the body that it's time to begin the incredible process of creating a new life. This hormone, produced by the cells that will eventually form the placenta, is responsible for maintaining the corpus luteum, which secretes progesterone to keep the uterine lining thick and hospitable for the embryo.

As the weeks progress, estrogen and progesterone levels rise dramatically. Progesterone, often referred to as the "pregnancy hormone," plays a critical role in relaxing the uterus muscles to prevent early contractions and stimulating the growth of blood vessels in the uterine lining to support the developing fetus. Estrogen, meanwhile, aids in the development of the placenta and stimulates the growth of the uterus itself.

Another key player is relaxin, a hormone that lives up to its name by relaxing the ligaments in the pelvis and softening and widening the cervix in preparation for childbirth. While its effects are most notable towards the end of pregnancy, relaxin begins to circulate early on. It is vital for the adjustments a woman's body must make to accommodate a growing baby.

The symphony of hormones during pregnancy also includes oxytocin, which is often associated with labor as it induces contractions of the uterus. However, its role extends beyond childbirth; oxytocin also fosters the bond between mother and child and plays a part in the milk ejection reflex during breastfeeding.

Pregnancy is a time of heightened sensitivity and responsiveness to hormonal signals; these are just a few key players. Each hormone has a specific and crucial role, ensuring that the environment within the womb is ideally suited to the needs of the developing fetus. The balance and levels of these hormones are meticulously regulated, as even the slightest deviation can affect the health and development of both mother and child.

As we delve deeper into the role of hormones in fetal development, we'll explore how these chemical messengers not only support the growth and nourishment of the fetus but also prepare the mother's body for the act of giving birth and the subsequent journey of motherhood.

The intricate dance of hormones during pregnancy is nothing short of miraculous, reflecting the body's innate wisdom in fostering new life.

The Role of Hormones in Fetal Development

As we delve into the intricate dance of hormones during the gestational journey, it's essential to understand their pivotal role in developing a new life. From the moment of conception, a woman's body becomes a finely tuned orchestra of hormones, each with a specific part to play in the symphony of fetal development.

The first and perhaps most renowned of these hormonal players is human chorionic gonadotropin (hCG). This hormone is the chemical beacon that signals a positive result on a pregnancy test. But its role extends far beyond that initial announcement. hCG ensures the corpus luteum—remnants of the follicle that released the egg—continues to secrete progesterone and estrogen, vital in maintaining the uterine lining and setting the stage for the embryo's implantation and nourishment.

Progesterone, often called the "pregnancy hormone," takes on the crucial task of keeping the uterine lining healthy and thick, creating a supportive environment for the embryo. It also relaxes the uterus muscles, preventing contractions that could disrupt the pregnancy. As the placenta grows, it takes over progesterone production, steadily increasing its levels to adapt to the fetus's needs.

Estrogen, another critical hormone, rises alongside progesterone. It stimulates blood flow to the womb and fosters the growth of the placenta, ensuring the fetus receives the oxygen and nutrients essential for development. Estrogen also plays a role in developing the breast's milk ducts, preparing the body for the nurturing phase post-birth.

The placenta, an organ unique to pregnancy, acts not only as a nourishment conduit but also as an endocrine powerhouse, producing various hormones that support fetal growth and prepare the mother's body for childbirth. One such hormone is human placental lactogen (hPL), which helps to regulate the mother's metabolism and ensures that the growing fetus has an adequate supply of nutrients.

As the fetus develops, its tiny endocrine system begins to shape. The fetal adrenal glands produce dehydroepiandrosterone (DHEA), which the placenta converts into estrogen, further supporting the pregnancy. The fetal thyroid gland also starts to function, producing thyroid hormones critical for brain development and growth regulation.

The interplay of these hormones is a delicate balance, a testament to the body's innate wisdom. Each hormonal shift is like a brushstroke in the masterpiece of human development, painting the picture of a new life in the womb's protective canvas.

Understanding the hormonal milieu of pregnancy not only highlights the marvel of life's beginnings but also underscores the importance of supporting hormonal health throughout this transformative period. As we move forward, we'll explore how to navigate and manage these hormonal fluctuations to foster a healthy pregnancy for both mother and child.

Managing Hormonal Fluctuations in Pregnancy

As it embarks on the pregnancy journey, the body becomes a symphony of hormones, each playing a vital role in supporting your health and the development of a child. Understanding and managing these hormonal fluctuations can help to create a smoother pregnancy experience.

Estrogen and progesterone are the stars of this hormonal ballet, rising steadily to create a nurturing environment for the baby. These hormones, while essential, can also stir up a whirlwind of changes in the body, affecting everything from your mood to your metabolism.

One of the most common experiences during pregnancy is the emotional rollercoaster that can come with these hormonal shifts. One might find themselves feeling joyous one moment and tearful the next, often without a clear trigger. This is perfectly normal, and giving yourself grace during these times is essential. Communicating openly with your partner, family, and friends about what you're going through can help them provide the support you need.

Physical symptoms like nausea, often referred to as morning sickness, can also be a byproduct of hormonal changes. While it's typically more pronounced during the first trimester, it can persist or come and go throughout pregnancy. Eating small, frequent meals and staying hydrated can help manage these symptoms. Ginger tea and acupressure wristbands are also natural remedies that some women find helpful.

As the body adapts to its new hormonal milieu, one might notice changes in their skin and hair. The 'pregnancy glow' is not a myth; it results from increased blood flow and oil production. However, this can also lead to acne or other skin changes. Using gentle, non-comedogenic skincare products can help maintain skin health. Similarly, while some women enjoy thicker, more lustrous hair during pregnancy, others might experience hair thinning or changes in texture. A balanced diet and proper hair care can mitigate these effects.

Sleep patterns can be disrupted by hormonal fluctuations as well. Progesterone, in particular, can make you feel more fatigued. Creating a calming bedtime routine and ensuring a comfortable sleeping environment can aid in better sleep. Don't hesitate to use pillows to support your changing body.

It's also essential to monitor and manage any hormonal-related health concerns, such as gestational diabetes or preeclampsia, with the guidance of a healthcare provider. Regular prenatal visits are crucial for tracking hormone levels and health during pregnancy.

Remember, while these hormonal changes are temporary, their impact on the body and mind can be significant. It's okay to seek help and advice, whether from healthcare professionals, support groups, or your personal network. Your well-being is as important as the healthy development of the baby, and taking care of yourself is the first step in taking care of your little one.

Keep in mind that each woman's experience with pregnancy is unique. What works for one may not work for another, so listening to your body and finding what brings you comfort and health is important. With understanding and care, you can manage these hormonal fluctuations and embrace the miracle of life unfolding within you.

Postpartum Hormonal Adjustments

As the journey of pregnancy culminates in the marvel of childbirth, a woman's body embarks on a new chapter of transformation. The postpartum period, often called the fourth trimester, is a time of immense hormonal shifts as the body transitions from pregnancy to its non-pregnant state. Understanding these hormonal adjustments can be helpful for new mothers navigating the postpartum period.

Immediately after delivery, the levels of pregnancy-related hormones such as estrogen and progesterone plummet. This sudden drop is a biological signal that you are no longer pregnant and triggers various physical and emotional responses. For instance, it's not uncommon for new mothers to experience a rollercoaster of emotions, often referred to as the "baby blues," which can include mood swings, weepiness, and feelings of overwhelm. These are typically short-lived, lasting a few days to a few weeks after delivery.

Another significant hormonal change involves the hormone prolactin, which rises during pregnancy and remains high if you are breastfeeding. Prolactin is responsible for milk production and affects mood and libido. Oxytocin, known as the love hormone, is also pivotal during this time. It facilitates bonding with your newborn and stimulates uterine contractions that help the uterus return to its pre-pregnancy size.

The thyroid gland can also be affected postpartum. Some women may experience postpartum thyroiditis, which can present with symptoms of both hyperthyroidism and hypothyroidism. This condition usually resolves independently, but it's important to be aware of the symptoms and seek medical advice if you suspect thyroid dysfunction.

It's essential to acknowledge that every woman's experience with postpartum hormonal adjustments is unique. While some may navigate this period relatively easily, others may find it more challenging. If you find yourself struggling with persistent mood changes, excessive fatigue, or other symptoms that concern you, it's important to reach out to your healthcare provider. Postpartum depression is a serious condition that affects many women and requires medical attention.

Remember that the body also adapts to a new normal during this time. Patience and self-care are key. Rest when you can, nourish your body with healthy foods, and don't hesitate to ask for support from loved ones or professionals. Your hormone levels will gradually stabilize, but giving yourself grace during this adjustment period is essential.

In the next part of our journey through hormone health, we'll explore the hormonal effects of breastfeeding, which not only nurtures a newborn but also continues to influence the postpartum hormonal landscape.

Breastfeeding and Hormonal Effects

As the journey of motherhood continues beyond the arrival of a child, the act of breastfeeding ushers in a new chapter of hormonal interplay that is as complex as it is beautiful. This natural process is not only about nourishment; it's a symphony of hormonal signals that fosters bonding, supports a baby's development, and subtly readies the body for potential future pregnancies.

A cascade of hormonal activity is triggered when a baby latches onto the breast. The primary hormones involved in breastfeeding are prolactin and oxytocin. Prolactin, often referred to as the 'milk-making hormone,' rises during pregnancy and reaches its peak after delivery. It is responsible for producing breast milk and ensures a steady supply for as long as you choose to nurse: each time a baby feeds, prolactin levels in the body rise, reinforcing the milk production cycle.

Oxytocin, fondly known as the 'love hormone,' plays a pivotal role in the let-down reflex – a critical response where the milk is released from the alveoli, tiny sacs within the breast, into the milk ducts where a nursing infant can access it. This hormone facilitates bonding between mother and child and has calming effects on both. The physical closeness and skin-to-skin contact during breastfeeding further enhance the release of oxytocin, strengthening the emotional connection and providing a sense of peace and contentment.

Breastfeeding also has a significant impact on the menstrual cycle and fertility. The high levels of prolactin suppress the release of the hormones required for ovulation. This natural suppression can lead to lactational amenorrhea, a period during which menstruation is absent, providing a form of natural, though not entirely reliable, contraception known as the Lactational Amenorrhea Method (LAM). It's important to note that the return of fertility can vary significantly among women, and ovulation can occur even before the first postpartum period, so additional forms of contraception should be considered if avoiding pregnancy is the goal.

The hormonal effects of breastfeeding extend beyond the immediate postpartum period. Nursing can influence the return to pre-pregnancy weight, as lactation burns additional calories. It may also confer long-term health benefits, such as a reduced risk of certain breast and ovarian cancers. These protective effects are thought to be linked to the hormonal changes induced by breastfeeding, including the extended periods of low estrogen levels associated with lactational amenorrhea.

It's essential to acknowledge that while breastfeeding is a natural process, it's not always easy. Hormonal fluctuations, alongside physical and emotional challenges, can sometimes make breastfeeding a complex journey. Some women may experience difficulties with milk supply, latch, or other issues that can lead to feelings of frustration or inadequacy. It's crucial to seek support from healthcare providers, lactation consultants, and breastfeeding support groups, as they can offer guidance and reassurance during this time.

In the grand landscape of hormone health for women, breastfeeding is a remarkable period where the body's innate wisdom shines through. It's a time of profound transformation, not only for the baby, who thrives on the nourishment and comfort provided but also for the mother, whose body continues to amaze with its ability to adapt and nurture life in its most tender stages.

Chapter Summary

- Hormonal changes during pregnancy are normal, and orchestrate the development of new life with precision and care.

- Understanding and managing hormonal fluctuations during pregnancy can help create a smoother experience, addressing emotional changes, physical symptoms, and sleep disruptions.
- Human chorionic gonadotropin (hCG) is one of the first hormones in pregnancy, maintaining the corpus luteum and supporting the uterine lining.
- Progesterone, the "pregnancy hormone," relaxes the uterus muscles and stimulates blood vessel growth, while estrogen aids placenta development and uterus growth.
- Relaxin softens the pelvis ligaments and cervix, and oxytocin induces labor contractions and fosters mother-child bonding.
- The placenta acts as an endocrine organ, producing hormones like human placental lactogen (hPL) to regulate the mother's metabolism and support fetal growth.
- Fetal adrenal glands and thyroid contribute to hormone production, influencing estrogen levels and critical development.
- Postpartum hormonal adjustments involve a drop in pregnancy hormones, changes in mood, and the continuation of prolactin and oxytocin for breastfeeding and bonding.

4

PERIMENOPAUSE AND MENOPAUSE: TRANSITIONING PHASES

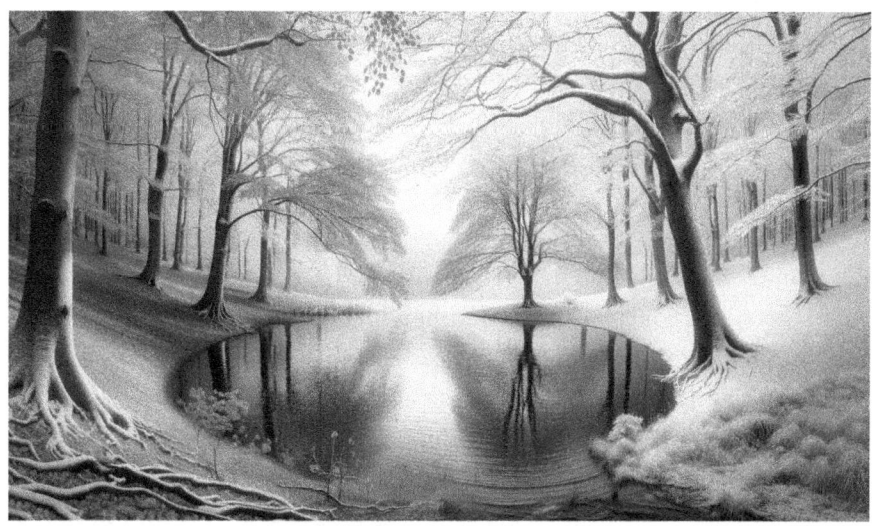

As the sun dips below the horizon, signaling the end of day and the beginning of twilight, so too does a woman's reproductive system signal its own transition. This natural shift is known as perimenopause. This term might be familiar, but its contours and nuances often remain shrouded in mystery. It's the prelude to a significant change when the body begins to compose a new narrative of hormone health.

Perimenopause typically commences in a woman's 40s, but for some, it can start as early as their 30s or as late as their 50s. It's a highly individual experience with a timeline spanning several years. During this phase, the ovaries gradually wind down their reproductive functions, producing less estrogen and progesterone—the hormones that have regulated menstruation and ovulation throughout a woman's life.

The ebb and flow of these hormones can be likened to the unpredictable patterns of the sea. Some days, the waters are calm, and on others, they are tumultuous. Women may notice that their menstrual cycles become irregular; periods may be heavier or lighter, longer or shorter, or they may skip a cycle entirely. This unpredictability is a hallmark of perimenopause and can be disconcerting. Still, it's important to remember that it's a normal part of the transition.

Beyond menstrual irregularity, other whispers of change may be felt. Some women experience hot flashes, those sudden waves of heat that wash over the body, often accompanied by a flushed face and sweating. Others might wake in the middle of the night, drenched in sweat—a nocturnal counterpart to hot flashes known as night sweats. These temperature irregularities are the body's response to the shifting sands of hormone levels.

Sleep disturbances during perimenopause are not limited to night sweats. The hormonal fluctuations can also lead to insomnia or restless sleep, making it difficult to get the restorative rest crucial to well-being. Mood swings may weave their way into daily life, with emotions swinging like a pendulum from joy to irritability or from energy to fatigue without a moment's notice.

It's not uncommon for women to notice changes in their sexual health during this time. Vaginal dryness and a decrease in libido can occur, which may affect intimacy and sexual relationships. These symptoms are rooted in the body's hormonal adjustments and are a normal part of the transition.

For some, perimenopause can also bring about a sense of loss or a challenge to their identity. The end of reproductive capability can evoke various emotions, from relief to sadness. It's important to acknowledge these feelings and understand that they are a natural response to change.

As we explore the waters of perimenopause, it's essential to remember that this is a time of transformation, not a disease to be cured. It's an opportunity to tune in to the body's signals and to care for oneself with compassion and understanding. Regular exercise, a balanced diet, stress management techniques, and open communication with healthcare providers and loved ones can all be part of a supportive strategy during this transition.

Perimenopause is the prelude to change, a time of preparation for the next stage of life's symphony. As we close this section, we carry with us the knowledge that while the body is shifting, it is also opening the door to a new phase of life—one that holds its unique beauty and challenges.

Understanding Menopause: Symptoms and Signs

As we navigate through the natural journey of hormonal shifts, understanding the signs and symptoms of menopause is like learning a new language spoken by our own bodies. This language, though at times seemingly foreign, is rich with information that can guide us toward self-care and informed choices.

Menopause, the cessation of menstruation for twelve consecutive months, is a natural biological process, not a medical condition. It marks the end of a woman's reproductive years, typically in the late 40s to early 50s. However, the experience of menopause is as unique as the individual, with symptoms varying widely in both type and intensity.

One of the most talked-about signs of menopause is the hot flash—a sudden warmth that spreads over the body, often most intense over the face, neck, and chest. These can be accompanied by sweating and sometimes followed by a chill. While the exact cause of hot flashes is not fully understood, they are thought to be related to the changes in hormone levels affecting the body's temperature regulation.

Night sweats, the nocturnal counterpart to hot flashes, can disrupt sleep and lead to insomnia. The importance of sleep for overall health cannot be overstated, so managing these symptoms is crucial. Many women find relief through lifestyle adjustments such as maintaining a cool sleeping environment and avoiding triggers like spicy foods or stress.

Irregular periods are another hallmark of the transition into menopause. You may notice changes in your menstrual cycle's frequency, duration, and flow. This unpredictability can be frustrating and sometimes alarming, but it's a normal part of the transition.

Vaginal dryness and discomfort during intercourse can occur as estrogen levels decline. These changes can affect sexual health and intimacy, but there are effective treatments and personal lubricants that can offer relief.

Emotional changes are also part of the menopause experience for many women. Mood swings, irritability, and feelings of sadness can be attributed to hormonal fluctuations, but they can also stem from the stress of dealing with other symptoms or life changes that often occur during this time.

Cognitive changes, such as difficulty concentrating and memory lapses, colloquially referred to as "menopause brain," can be concerning. It's important to note that these symptoms are usually temporary and can be mitigated through various strategies, including mental exercises and stress reduction techniques.

Physical changes are also evident during menopause. Many women experience a slowing metabolism and changes in weight distribution, often leading to weight gain around the abdomen. Maintaining a healthy diet and regular exercise routine can help manage these changes.

It's also a time to pay closer attention to bone health, as declining estrogen levels can decrease bone density, increasing the risk of osteoporosis. Calcium, vitamin D intake, and weight-bearing exercises are important preventive measures.

While these symptoms can be challenging, they are a natural part of the aging process. It's essential to approach this phase with self-compassion and to seek support from healthcare providers, friends, and family. Remember, menopause is not an end but a transition to a new phase of life that can be embraced with grace and resilience.

Hormone Replacement Therapy: Pros and Cons

As we navigate the transformative journey of perimenopause and menopause, many women consider various strategies to manage the symptoms that accompany these natural phases of life. One of the most discussed options is Hormone Replacement Therapy (HRT), which aims to replenish the body with estrogen and, in some cases, progesterone, which are no longer being produced at the levels they once were. The decision to use HRT is highly personal. It should be made with a thorough understanding of its potential benefits and risks.

On the positive side, HRT has been shown to be highly effective in alleviating some of the most common and uncomfortable symptoms of menopause, such as hot flashes, night sweats, vaginal dryness, and mood swings. By restoring hormone levels, HRT can also help prevent bone loss and reduce the risk of osteoporosis, a significant concern for many women as they age. Additionally, some studies suggest that HRT may offer some protection against heart disease when started early in the postmenopausal period.

However, the use of HRT is not without its controversies and potential drawbacks. The most significant concerns arise from studies that have linked the long-term use of certain types of HRT to an increased risk of breast cancer, blood clots, stroke, and heart disease. It's important to note that the risk varies depending on individual health factors, the type of hormones used, and the duration of therapy. For some women, particularly those with a family history of these conditions, the risks of HRT may outweigh the benefits.

Another consideration is the timing and duration of HRT. Research indicates that the window of opportunity for the potential benefits of HRT, particularly concerning heart health, may be limited to the early years of menopause. Furthermore, the current medical consensus generally recommends using the lowest effective dose for the shortest period necessary to manage symptoms.

It's also essential to recognize that HRT is not a one-size-fits-all solution. Women's bodies and responses to hormonal changes are as unique as their life stories. Therefore, the decision to use HRT should be made in close consultation with a healthcare provider, taking into account personal health history, family history, lifestyle, and the severity of menopausal symptoms.

For those who are candidates for HRT, there are various forms available, including pills, patches, gels, and creams. Each method has pros and cons, and what works for one woman may not be the best choice for another. It's a process of personalization and, sometimes, trial and error to find the most suitable and effective form of therapy.

In conclusion, while HRT can be a powerful tool in the management of menopausal symptoms and the prevention of specific long-term health issues, it is not a decision to be taken lightly. It requires a thoughtful conversation with a healthcare provider, a clear understanding of personal health risks, and a commitment to ongoing monitoring and adjustment. For those who decide that HRT is not the right choice or for those seeking complementary strategies, there are natural approaches to managing menopausal symptoms that can also offer relief and support during this phase of life.

Natural Approaches to Menopausal Symptoms

As we navigate the journey of perimenopause and menopause, it's essential to acknowledge that each woman's experience is as unique as she is. While hormone replacement therapy (HRT) has been discussed as one option for managing symptoms, many women seek natural approaches to find relief and support their bodies during this transition. Let's explore some natural strategies that can help ease the menopausal journey.

Lifestyle modifications are often the first line of defense. Regular physical activity is not only good for your heart and bones. Still, it can also help reduce hot flashes and improve mood. Aim for at least 150 minutes of moderate aerobic activity per week, complemented by strength training exercises. Yoga and tai chi, in particular, can be beneficial for stress reduction and improving balance, which can be affected during menopause.

The diet also plays a crucial role in managing menopausal symptoms. Foods rich in phytoestrogens, such as soybeans, flaxseeds, and certain whole grains, may offer a natural way to balance hormones. These plant-based compounds can mimic the effects of estrogen in the body, potentially easing hot flashes and other symptoms. However, it's essential to consult with a healthcare provider before making significant dietary changes, especially if you have any underlying health conditions.

Hydration is another crucial element. As simple as it sounds, drinking enough water can help with bloating and the dryness that often accompanies menopause. Aim for eight glasses daily, and consider adding hydrating foods like cucumbers and watermelon to your diet.

Sleep can become elusive during menopause, with night sweats and insomnia being common complaints. Creating a sleep-conducive environment, maintaining a regular bedtime routine, and possibly incorporating relaxation techniques like meditation or deep breathing exercises can be helpful. Some women find relief in natural supplements like melatonin, but it's important to discuss this with a healthcare provider before starting any new supplement regimen.

Herbal remedies have been used for centuries to alleviate menopausal symptoms. Herbs such as black cohosh, red clover, and dong quai are popular. Still, scientific evidence on their effectiveness varies, and they can interact with medications. Always consult with a healthcare professional before trying herbal treatments.

Stress management is also vital. Chronic stress can exacerbate menopausal symptoms, so finding effective ways to relax and decompress is essential. Mindfulness, therapy, or simply carving out time for hobbies and activities you enjoy can make a significant difference in your overall well-being.

Lastly, social support cannot be underestimated. Connecting with other women who are going through similar experiences can provide comfort and valuable insights. Whether through support groups, online forums, or just chatting with friends, sharing your journey can be incredibly therapeutic.

Remember, these natural approaches aim not just to treat symptoms but to enhance overall health and quality of life during menopause. It's about finding what works for you and making adjustments as needed, always in consultation with healthcare professionals who understand your health history and needs.

As we continue to explore the facets of hormone health for women, it's clear that the interplay between hormones and various aspects of health is complex. Next, we'll delve into the relationship between hormones and bone health, a critical consideration for aging women who want to maintain strength and vitality through menopause.

Bone Health and Hormones in Aging Women

As we gracefully navigate the waves of perimenopause and menopause, it's crucial to shine a light on an aspect of our health that often goes unnoticed until it demands our attention: our bones. Bone health is a silent but significant concern for aging women, and it's intimately tied to the hormonal changes that occur during this time.

Our bones are living tissues that constantly break down and rebuild. This process is regulated by hormones, including estrogen, which plays a pivotal role in maintaining bone density. During the fertile years, estrogen helps keep bone breakdown and rebuilding in balance. However, as we approach perimenopause and transition into menopause, estrogen levels begin to fluctuate and ultimately decline. This decline can accelerate bone loss, increasing the risk of osteoporosis—a condition where bones become weak and brittle.

Understanding the connection between hormones and bone health is the first step in taking proactive measures to protect and strengthen our skeletal framework. It's not just about preventing fractures; it's about maintaining a quality of life that allows us to continue the activities we love and live without the fear of injury.

So, what can we do to support our bone health during these years of change? Nutrition is a cornerstone. A diet rich in calcium and vitamin D is essential for bone strength. Calcium is a building block for bones, while vitamin D helps our bodies absorb calcium effectively. However, it's not just about the intake of these nutrients; it's also about how well our bodies can utilize them. Factors such as vitamin K2 and magnesium also play roles in bone health, helping to ensure calcium is deposited in our bones rather than in other tissues that can cause harm.

Physical activity, particularly weight-bearing and resistance exercises, is another powerful tool in our bone health arsenal. These activities improve strength and balance, reduce the risk of falls, and stimulate bone formation. Even simple activities like walking, dancing, or lifting weights can make a significant difference.

For some women, hormone replacement therapy (HRT) may be a consideration to help mitigate bone loss. It's a decision that should be made in close consultation with a healthcare provider, weighing the benefits against potential risks. HRT isn't suitable for everyone, but it can be an effective part of a comprehensive bone health strategy for certain individuals.

Addressing lifestyle factors that can negatively impact bone health is important. Smoking and excessive alcohol consumption can both contribute to bone loss, so taking steps to quit smoking and moderate alcohol intake can be beneficial. Additionally, being mindful of medications that may affect bone density, such as long-term use of steroids, is essential.

Lastly, regular screenings can play a critical role in maintaining bone health. Bone density tests, such as DEXA scans, can help detect osteoporosis before a fracture occurs, allowing for early intervention. These screenings are crucial for women with risk factors for osteoporosis, such as a family history of the condition, a petite body frame, or certain medical conditions and treatments.

The transition through perimenopause and menopause calls for a renewed commitment to our overall well-being, with bone health being a vital component. By understanding the hormonal shifts that occur and their impact on our bones, we can take informed and practical steps to ensure that our skeletal health supports us as we move through these chapters of life with strength and vitality.

Chapter Summary

- Perimenopause marks the beginning of the transition in a woman's reproductive system, typically starting in the 40s but can vary widely.
- During perimenopause, ovaries produce less estrogen and progesterone, leading to irregular menstrual cycles and symptoms like hot flashes and night sweats.
- Women may experience sleep disturbances, mood swings, and changes in sexual health, including vaginal dryness and decreased libido. The transition can evoke various emotions, from relief to sadness, as women come to terms with the end of their reproductive years.
- Menopause is the cessation of menstruation for twelve consecutive months, usually occurring in the late 40s to early 50s, with widespread symptoms.
- Common menopause symptoms include hot flashes, night sweats, irregular periods, vaginal dryness, emotional changes, cognitive challenges, and physical changes like weight gain.
- Hormone Replacement Therapy can alleviate menopausal symptoms and prevent bone loss but carries risks such as increased chances of breast cancer and heart disease.
- Natural approaches to managing menopausal symptoms include lifestyle changes, diet, hydration, sleep management, herbal remedies, stress management, and social support.
- Bone health is crucial during perimenopause and menopause due to declining estrogen levels, with nutrition and physical activity vital to maintaining bone density.
- Hormone Replacement Therapy may be considered for bone health. Lifestyle factors like smoking and alcohol consumption should be managed, and regular bone density screenings are recommended.

5

THYROID HEALTH: THE METABOLIC REGULATOR

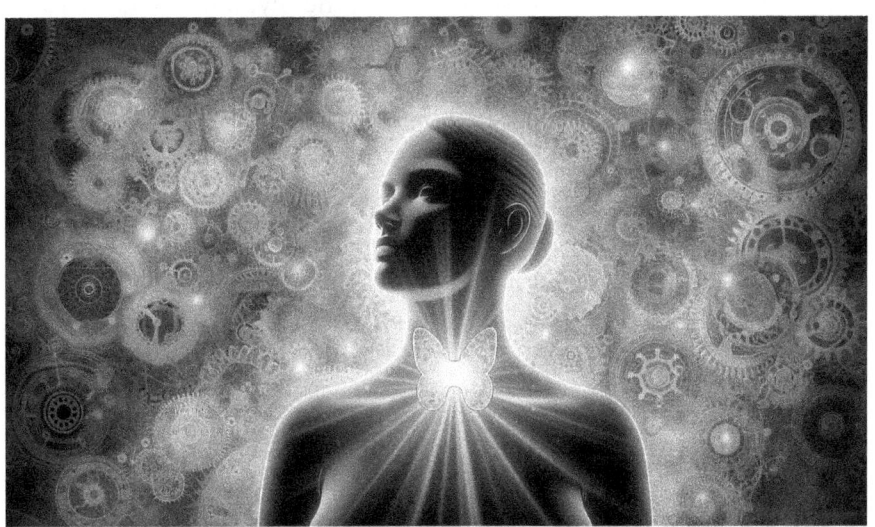

N estled at the base of your neck, the thyroid gland may be small, but its impact on your body is mighty. This butterfly-shaped gland is the maestro of your metabolism, conducting the symphony of hormones that regulate how your body uses energy. Understanding how your thyroid functions is like uncovering the secret to how your body's cells dance to the rhythm of life.

The thyroid produces two main hormones: thyroxine (T4) and triiodothyronine (T3). These hormones travel through your bloodstream and reach nearly every cell, influencing multiple functions such as your heart rate, body temperature, and how quickly you burn calories. It's a delicate balance, and when it's just right, you feel like you're on top of the world—energized, focused, and balanced.

But what happens when this balance is disrupted? Imagine a car with a sputtering engine or a clock that ticks too slowly. That's akin to what your body experiences when the thyroid isn't producing enough hormones—a condition known as hypothyroidism. It's like the conductor of your metabolic orchestra has suddenly slowed the tempo, and every musician (or cell) is struggling to keep up.

The thyroid's ability to produce these vital hormones hinges on a complex feedback loop involving the hypothalamus and the pituitary gland, two key players in your brain. The hypothalamus releases thyrotropin-releasing hormone (TRH), which prompts the pituitary gland to produce thyroid-stimulating hormone (TSH). TSH then signals to the thyroid how much T4 and T3 should be released into the bloodstream. It's a finely tuned system; when it works well, it's seamless and unnoticeable. But when it doesn't, the effects on your body and well-being can be profound.

For women, maintaining thyroid health is particularly crucial. The ebb and flow of female hormones can influence thyroid function, and various stages of a woman's life—such as puberty, pregnancy, and menopause—can change thyroid hormone levels. It's not uncommon for women to first notice symptoms of a thyroid imbalance during these times of hormonal fluctuation.

So, how do you know if your thyroid is not performing its role as it should? It starts with tuning into your body and recognizing the signs that may indicate your thyroid is underactive. In the next section, we'll delve into hypothyroidism, exploring what happens when your thyroid slows down, the symptoms to watch for, and how this condition can affect your overall health. It's a journey into understanding the subtler aspects of your body's internal workings, and with knowledge comes the power to seek harmony within.

Hypothyroidism: When the Thyroid Slows Down

In the intricate dance of hormones that governs our well-being, the thyroid gland plays a pivotal role, orchestrating many bodily functions with the precision of a seasoned conductor. When this gland's activity diminishes, a condition known as hypothyroidism emerges, casting a wide net over one's health and vitality.

Hypothyroidism is akin to a slow-burning flame, often starting so subtly that it's easily dismissed or mistaken for the wear and tear of daily life. Women, in particular, may notice a gradual onset of fatigue that no amount of sleep seems to alleviate. It's as if the body's internal battery is perpetually low, no matter how long it's been on charge.

But fatigue is just the tip of the iceberg. With hypothyroidism, the metabolism—the body's engine for burning calories—downshifts. Weight gain may occur, even when eating habits haven't changed. The skin, once supple, may become dry and cool to the touch, while hair that was once lustrous and full may turn brittle and thin. These physical changes are not merely cosmetic but external manifestations of an internal imbalance.

The thyroid's influence extends to the very rhythm of our hearts. A slower heartbeat can be a sign of an underactive thyroid, as can an increase in blood cholesterol levels, which is why hypothyroidism is often discovered during routine health screenings.

For women, the menstrual cycle is a delicate interplay of hormones, and the thyroid is a key player. An underactive thyroid can lead to heavier, more frequent, and more painful periods. It can also be a stealthy saboteur of fertility, often overlooked in the quest to conceive.

The mental and emotional realms are not immune to the thyroid's reach. Hypothyroidism can cloud the mind, making concentration difficult and memory elusive. It can also cast a shadow over one's mood, contributing to feelings of depression or a pervasive sense of malaise.

Diagnosing hypothyroidism involves a careful evaluation of symptoms and blood tests that measure thyroid hormone levels. The most common treatment is a daily dose of synthetic thyroid hormone, which replaces what the body can no longer produce in sufficient quantities.

This medication, typically a lifelong commitment, is a beacon of hope for many, often restoring energy levels and normalizing bodily functions.

Living with hypothyroidism is a journey of balance and awareness. It requires tuning in to the body's signals and working closely with healthcare providers to fine-tune treatment. It's about understanding that this small gland, nestled in the neck, holds great power over the symphony of hormones that animate our lives.

As we navigate the complexities of hormone health, it's essential to remember that each person's experience with hypothyroidism is unique. Patience and self-compassion become vital companions on the path to wellness, reminding us that the journey is as much about nurturing the spirit as it is about treating the body.

Hyperthyroidism: The Overactive Thyroid

In the intricate dance of hormones that governs our well-being, the thyroid gland often takes center stage, especially for women. When it becomes overactive—a condition known as hyperthyroidism—it can lead to a symphony of symptoms that disrupt the rhythm of daily life.

Hyperthyroidism occurs when the thyroid gland produces too much of the hormones thyroxine (T4) and triiodothyronine (T3). Excessive amounts of these hormones accelerate bodily functions, leading to various signs and symptoms.

Imagine your body as a car. With hyperthyroidism, it's as if the thyroid is pushing the accelerator too hard. You might experience a rapid or irregular heartbeat, a sensation that your heart is pounding (palpitations), and even the feeling of being on edge or nervous. These are the telltale signs that your body is running on overdrive.

Weight loss is another familiar hallmark of hyperthyroidism, even when your appetite and food intake remain the same or increase. It can be puzzling and distressing to lose weight without trying, and it's often what prompts many women to seek medical advice. Alongside this, you may notice increased sweating, sensitivity to heat, and a more frequent need to quench your thirst.

For women, menstrual cycles can become lighter and less frequent.

This disruption to the menstrual cycle is not only a concern for overall health but can also affect fertility. It reminds us how closely our reproductive health is linked to proper thyroid functioning.

Changes in mood and mental state can accompany the physical changes. You might feel unusually anxious, irritable, or having difficulty concentrating. Sleep can become elusive despite feeling tired, creating a frustrating cycle of fatigue and restlessness.

In some cases, you may notice a swelling at the base of your neck, which is a goiter. This is the thyroid gland becoming enlarged and can be a visual clue that something is amiss. While not all cases of hyperthyroidism result in noticeable goiters, their presence can exacerbate the feeling of tightness or discomfort in the throat, sometimes making swallowing a challenge.

The causes of hyperthyroidism are varied, with autoimmune disorders, nodules on the thyroid gland, and certain medications being among the common culprits. Understanding the underlying cause is crucial for effective treatment, which may include medication to reduce hormone production, radioactive iodine to shrink the gland, or even surgery in some cases.

Living with hyperthyroidism can be a delicate balancing act, requiring careful monitoring and often lifelong management. It's a journey that can sometimes feel overwhelming. Still, with the proper support and treatment, many women find a new equilibrium. The key is to listen to your body, advocate for your health, and work closely with healthcare professionals who understand the nuances of thyroid disorders.

As we navigate the complexities of thyroid health, it's important to remember that each woman's experience is unique. Whether you're dealing with the slowing down of hypothyroidism or the acceleration of hyperthyroidism, your story is your own. And while the path to managing thyroid conditions is not always straightforward, it's a path that leads to a deeper understanding of your body and its needs.

Autoimmune Thyroid Diseases: Hashimoto's and Graves'

The thyroid gland plays a pivotal role in orchestrating various metabolic processes in the intricate dance of the body's endocrine system. For many women, the harmony of this dance is disrupted by autoimmune thyroid diseases, which can lead to a cascade of health challenges. Two of the most common conditions are Hashimoto's thyroiditis and Graves' disease, each representing opposite ends of the thyroid function spectrum.

Hashimoto's thyroiditis is the most prevalent form of thyroid inflammation. It is often the underlying cause of hypothyroidism, a state in which the thyroid gland underproduces hormones. This condition is characterized by the immune system mistakenly attacking the thyroid, leading to damage and impaired hormone production. Women with Hashimoto's may experience a variety of symptoms, including fatigue, weight gain, cold intolerance, and muscle weakness, among others. The onset of Hashimoto's is typically gradual, and it may take years before the symptoms prompt a woman to seek medical attention.

Conversely, Graves' disease is an autoimmune disorder that leads to hyperthyroidism or an overactive thyroid. In Graves' disease, the immune system produces antibodies that bind to the thyroid gland, causing it to produce an excess of thyroid hormones. This overactivity can manifest in symptoms such as unexplained weight loss, rapid heartbeat, increased sweating, and anxiety. Unlike the slow progression of Hashimoto's, the symptoms of Graves' disease can emerge more abruptly. They can be more immediately disruptive to a woman's well-being.

Diagnosing these conditions typically involves a combination of blood tests to measure thyroid hormone levels and the presence of specific antibodies, along with a thorough clinical evaluation. Imaging studies like ultrasound or radioactive iodine uptake tests may also be employed to understand the thyroid's structure and function better.

Management of Hashimoto's and Graves' disease often requires a personalized approach, as the impact on each woman's body can vary greatly. For those with Hashimoto's, treatment usually involves hormone replacement therapy to restore normal thyroid hormone levels. In the case of Graves' disease, treatment options may include medications to inhibit hormone production, radioactive iodine therapy to reduce thyroid activity, or surgery in more severe cases.

Living with an autoimmune thyroid disease can be an emotional journey, as the symptoms can affect not only physical health but also emotional well-being and quality of life. It's important for women to have a supportive healthcare team that not only addresses the physiological aspects of the disease but also provides guidance on coping with the emotional and psychological impacts.

As we move forward, understanding the role of nutrition and lifestyle in supporting thyroid health becomes increasingly important. While medical treatments address physiological imbalances, integrating holistic practices can empower women to manage their condition and improve their overall well-being actively.

Nutrition and Lifestyle for Thyroid Health

In the intricate dance of hormones that governs a woman's health, the thyroid plays a pivotal role, orchestrating the tempo at which her body operates. The right nutrition and lifestyle choices can be influential conductors for this metabolic symphony, helping to maintain harmony and balance.

A well-rounded diet is essential when nourishing the thyroid, starting with the basics. This means embracing a variety of fruits and vegetables, which are rich in antioxidants and essential nutrients. These colorful foods are not just a feast for the eyes; they provide the vitamins and minerals your thyroid needs to function optimally.

Among these nutrients, iodine is a critical component for thyroid hormone production. While iodine deficiency is less common in many developed countries due to iodized salt, it's still important to include natural sources in your diet. Seaweed, fish, and dairy are excellent sources of iodine. Still, consuming them in moderation is vital to avoid an excess, which can be just as detrimental as a deficiency.

Selenium is another mineral that deserves a spotlight. It plays a crucial role in the conversion of thyroid hormones from their inactive to active forms. Foods like Brazil nuts, sunflower seeds, and whole grains are rich in selenium and can support thyroid health.

But it's not just about what you eat; it's also about how you eat. Stress can wreak havoc on your thyroid, and one way to combat this is through mindful eating. Taking the time to savor your food, eating slowly, and listening to your body's hunger cues can help manage stress levels and support overall well-being.

Physical activity is another cornerstone of a thyroid-friendly lifestyle. Regular exercise can help regulate thyroid function, boost mood, and improve energy levels. It doesn't have to be a high-intensity workout; even a daily walk or gentle yoga can make a significant difference.

Sleep, that often-neglected aspect of health, is also vital for thyroid function. Aim for 7-9 hours of quality sleep per night. Establishing a calming bedtime routine and ensuring your bedroom is a sanctuary can help you drift off to the restorative sleep your body—and thyroid—needs.

Lastly, avoiding certain substances that can interfere with thyroid function is important. Smoking, excessive alcohol consumption, and exposure to environmental toxins can all harm thyroid health. Being mindful of these factors and minimizing exposure can benefit your thyroid and overall health.

Remember, each woman's body is unique, and what works for one may not work for another. It's always wise to consult with a healthcare provider before significantly changing your diet or lifestyle, especially if you have a thyroid condition. They can provide personalized advice that takes into account your individual health needs.

By embracing these nutritional and lifestyle practices, you're not just supporting your thyroid but investing in your overall health and well-being. It's a journey of self-care that can lead to a more vibrant, balanced life.

Chapter Summary

- The thyroid gland, located at the base of the neck, is crucial for metabolism, producing hormones T4 and T3 that affect energy use in the body.
- Women's thyroid health is vital due to hormonal fluctuations during puberty, pregnancy, and menopause.
- Thyroid hormone imbalances can lead to hypothyroidism, where the body's functions slow down, or hyperthyroidism, where they speed up.
- Hypothyroidism symptoms include fatigue, weight gain, dry skin, slow heart rate, menstrual changes, and mental fog, and it's treated with synthetic hormones.
- Hyperthyroidism symptoms include rapid heartbeat, weight loss, heat sensitivity, menstrual changes, and anxiety, and it's treated with medication, radioactive iodine, or surgery.
- Autoimmune thyroid diseases like Hashimoto's thyroiditis (leading to hypothyroidism) and Graves' disease (leading to hyperthyroidism) affect the thyroid's function.
- Nutrition and lifestyle choices, such as a balanced diet rich in iodine and selenium, mindful eating, regular exercise, and adequate sleep, support thyroid health.
- Avoiding substances that interfere with thyroid function, like smoking and environmental toxins, is vital for maintaining thyroid and overall health.

6

STRESS AND HORMONES: THE ADRENAL CONNECTION

In the intricate dance of the body's response to stress, understanding the physiology is like learning the steps to a complex routine. It's a choreography that involves various organs and hormones, all working in tandem to help you navigate through the challenges that life throws your way.

The adrenal gland is at the heart of this dance, a small but mighty organ that sits atop your kidneys like a hat. When you encounter a stressful situation, your brain sends a signal to these glands, cueing them to release a cascade of hormones. These hormones are the body's equivalent of a backstage crew working behind the scenes to prepare you for action.

The initial response is almost instantaneous. Adrenaline, also known as epinephrine, floods your system, heightening your senses, quickening your pulse, and pumping more blood to your muscles. This is the 'fight or flight' response that our ancestors relied on for survival, and it's just as relevant today when we need to react swiftly to a potential threat or challenge.

But the stress response doesn't end there. After the initial surge of adrenaline, the adrenals release another hormone that plays a longer-term role in how your body manages stress. This hormone is cortisol, often referred to as the stress hormone, and it has a wide range of effects on your body.

Cortisol ensures that your body has enough energy to deal with prolonged stress. It does this by increasing glucose in the bloodstream, enhancing your brain's use of glucose, and increasing the availability of substances that repair tissues. Cortisol also curbs functions that would be nonessential or detrimental in a fight-or-flight situation. It alters immune system responses and suppresses the digestive system, the reproductive system, and growth processes.

This complex hormonal interplay is designed to be self-regulating. Once the perceived threat has passed, hormone levels should return to normal as part of the body's feedback mechanism. However, this system can become overtaxed in our modern world with its constant barrage of stressors. When stress becomes chronic, the adrenal glands may continue to produce cortisol at elevated levels. This can lead to a host of issues, as the body is constantly alert, never quite returning to its baseline.

Understanding the physiology of stress is crucial because it helps us recognize the importance of managing our stress response. It's not just about feeling less frazzled; it's about maintaining the delicate balance of our hormonal health. As we move forward, we'll delve deeper into cortisol, the stress hormone, and explore its profound impact on our bodies and well-being.

Cortisol: The Stress Hormone

In the intricate dance of hormones that affects every aspect of a woman's health, cortisol plays a lead role in stress. Often referred to as the "stress hormone," cortisol is produced by the adrenal glands, which are small but mighty organs perched atop your kidneys like vigilant sentinels. Understanding cortisol's function is crucial to comprehending how stress influences our bodies and, more specifically, its unique implications for women.

Cortisol is not a villain. In fact, it's essential for survival. It helps regulate various processes in the body, including metabolism and the immune response. It also has a pivotal role in helping the body respond to stress. When you encounter a stressful situation, your brain triggers the release of cortisol. This hormone then courses through your body, preparing you for the "fight or flight" response. It sharpens your senses, quickens your heartbeat, and releases energy stores to give you the necessary resources to handle the challenge at hand.

However, the story of cortisol is a tale of balance. While acute stress can lead to a temporary spike in cortisol, which is normal and often beneficial, the problems arise when stress becomes chronic. In today's fast-paced world, many women find themselves in a constant state of low-grade stress, whether it's due to work pressures, family responsibilities, health concerns, or social dynamics. This persistent stress can lead to a sustained high level of cortisol, which is where the trouble begins.

High cortisol levels over prolonged periods can adversely affect your health. It can disrupt sleep, lead to weight gain, increase blood pressure, and contribute to mood swings or feelings of anxiety. These effects can be particularly pronounced for women due to the interplay between cortisol and female sex hormones like estrogen and progesterone.

Moreover, the impact of sustained high cortisol can extend to menstrual cycles, potentially causing irregular periods or worsening symptoms of premenstrual syndrome (PMS). It can also play a role in the onset of menopause and the severity of its symptoms. During menopause, as the body's production of estrogen and progesterone decreases, the sensitivity to cortisol can increase, making stress management even more critical.

It's essential to recognize the signs that your body may be experiencing the adverse effects of too much cortisol. These can include fatigue, difficulty concentrating, and a general sense of being overwhelmed. By acknowledging these signals, you can take proactive steps to manage stress and, in turn, help regulate your cortisol levels.

Several strategies can help maintain healthy cortisol levels. Regular physical activity is one of the most effective, as it can boost mood and improve sleep, which can help modulate cortisol production. Mindfulness practices, such as meditation or deep breathing exercises, can be beneficial. Maintaining a balanced diet and ensuring adequate rest are critical components of a holistic approach to managing stress and supporting hormone health.

In essence, cortisol is a critical hormone that helps your body cope with stress but requires a delicate balance. Too much or too little can have significant implications for your overall well-being. Understanding cortisol's role and taking steps to manage stress can support your body's natural rhythms and promote hormone health, an essential part of a balanced and healthy life as a woman.

Adrenal Fatigue: Myth or Reality?

In the bustling rhythm of modern life, where stress often seems like a constant companion, the term "adrenal fatigue" has found a foothold in conversations about health and well-being, particularly among women. It's a phrase used to describe a collection of symptoms believed to be caused by a prolonged, overactive stress response that eventually wears down the adrenal glands, leading to exhaustion.

Recall that the small but mighty adrenal glands sit atop your kidneys like vigilant sentinels, orchestrating your body's reactions to stress through the release of hormones such as cortisol, which we've explored in depth. When life's demands become relentless, these glands are put through their paces, pumping out these hormones to help you navigate the challenges you face.

But what happens when the stress is unending when the alarm bells of your life never seem to quiet? This is where the concept of adrenal fatigue enters the conversation. It suggests that after long periods of chronic stress, the adrenal glands can no longer keep up with the body's demand for these regulatory hormones, leading to symptoms such as fatigue, sleep disturbances, weight gain, and a craving for salt or sugar.

However, it's important to approach this topic with a discerning eye. The medical community is divided on the existence of adrenal fatigue as a medical diagnosis. Conventional medicine does recognize conditions such as Addison's disease, where the adrenal glands produce insufficient hormones, and Cushing's syndrome, characterized by an overproduction. Yet, adrenal fatigue occupies a gray area, with many health professionals questioning its validity due to a lack of robust scientific evidence.

Despite this skepticism in some circles, there are countless women who identify with the symptoms attributed to adrenal fatigue. They seek answers and relief for their persistent tiredness and other related health concerns. It's essential to validate these experiences, acknowledging that while the term "adrenal fatigue" may not be widely accepted, the symptoms are very real to those suffering from them.

In navigating this complex issue, it's crucial to consider the physiological and psychological components of stress. The body's response to stress is intricate. It can affect various systems beyond the adrenals, including the digestive, immune, and nervous systems. Therefore, addressing stress-related symptoms often requires a holistic approach that looks at lifestyle, diet, sleep, exercise, and emotional well-being.

For those feeling the weight of these symptoms, the journey toward balance and health can be a personal one, filled with trial and error. It involves tuning into your body's signals, recognizing when to slow down, and finding strategies that help restore your sense of equilibrium. This journey is not about chasing a one-size-fits-all solution but discovering what works for your unique body and situation.

As we move forward, we'll delve into practical strategies that can help manage stress and support hormonal balance. These approaches aim to empower you with tools to enhance your resilience against the pressures of life, fostering a sense of well-being that is both sustainable and nurturing.

Strategies for Managing Stress and Hormonal Balance

Stress is often the leader in the intricate dance of hormone health, guiding the tempo and rhythm of our hormonal responses. Understanding this, we can choreograph a life-supporting balance and well-being. Let's explore strategies to help manage stress and maintain hormonal harmony.

First and foremost, nurturing a healthy diet is paramount. Foods rich in vitamins and minerals, such as leafy greens, nuts, seeds, and lean proteins, provide the nutrients necessary for adrenal support. Integrating complex carbohydrates like whole grains can help stabilize blood sugar levels, supporting adrenal health. Additionally, certain herbs such as ashwagandha and rhodiola have been traditionally used to help the body adapt to stress.

Regular physical activity is another cornerstone of stress management. Exercise not only helps to reduce the levels of stress hormones in the body but also boosts the production of endorphins, the body's natural mood elevators. Whether it's a brisk walk, a yoga session, or a dance class, finding an activity that brings joy can make exercise an enjoyable and effective stress reliever.

Mindfulness and relaxation techniques such as meditation, deep breathing exercises, and progressive muscle relaxation can also help manage stress. These practices help calm the mind and reduce the physiological effects of stress, promoting a sense of tranquility that supports hormonal balance.

Sleep is an often underestimated yet crucial component of hormonal health. Establishing a regular sleep routine and creating a restful environment can enhance the quality of sleep, which in turn can help regulate the production and release of stress hormones.

Lastly, fostering strong social connections and seeking support can provide emotional comfort and reduce stress. Whether talking with a friend, joining a support group, or seeking professional counseling, having a network to lean on is invaluable.

By incorporating these strategies into daily life, it's possible to create a foundation supporting hormonal health and overall well-being. Remember, the journey to balance is personal and unique to each individual. It's about finding what works for you and making small, sustainable changes that can lead to a healthier, more harmonious life.

Stress and Female Hormonal Disorders

Stress often steps on the toes of hormonal harmony, particularly for women. When stress enters the scene, the adrenal glands spring into action, secreting cortisol, the primary stress hormone. This response is part of the body's natural survival mechanism, the fight-or-flight response, which, in ancient times, was a crucial reaction to immediate threats.

However, the persistent stress of modern life doesn't come in the form of occasional predators but rather as a relentless stream of deadlines, social pressures, and multitasking demands. This constant state of alert can lead to an overproduction of cortisol, which, over time, can wreak havoc on the female body.

Cortisol's role is not inherently evil; it's essential for various bodily functions, including regulating metabolism, reducing inflammation, and assisting with memory formulation. But when stress is chronic, the sustained high levels of cortisol can lead to a cascade of female hormonal disorders.

One of the most significant impacts of prolonged stress is on the menstrual cycle. Cortisol can inhibit the production of gonadotropin-releasing hormone (GnRH), which is responsible for the release of the hormones that trigger ovulation and menstruation. This disruption can lead to irregular periods, anovulation, or even amenorrhea, the absence of menstruation.

Stress can also exacerbate premenstrual syndrome (PMS) and premenstrual dysphoric disorder (PMDD), conditions that affect a significant number of women. The delicate balance between estrogen and progesterone can be tipped by the scales of stress, leading to mood swings, bloating, and other symptoms that can range from mildly irritating to severely debilitating.

Furthermore, the relationship between stress and hormones extends to fertility. Chronic stress can impact fertility by affecting the hormones that are essential for conception. It can also influence libido, creating a challenging cycle for women who are trying to conceive, as stress about fertility can further impair hormonal balance and reproductive function.

The adrenal glands' overexertion doesn't stop with reproductive hormones. There's a complex interplay between cortisol and insulin, the hormone responsible for regulating blood sugar levels. High cortisol can lead to increased blood sugar, which, over time, can contribute to insulin resistance and the risk of developing type 2 diabetes.

Moreover, the adrenal glands' production of another hormone, DHEA (dehydroepiandrosterone), can be affected by stress. DHEA is involved in producing other hormones, including estrogen and testosterone. An imbalance in DHEA levels can lead to various symptoms, including fatigue, muscle loss, and decreased bone density, which are particularly concerning for women as they age.

The impact of stress on thyroid function is another critical aspect of the adrenal connection. The thyroid gland, which regulates metabolism, can be slowed down by high cortisol levels, leading to symptoms such as weight gain, fatigue, and depression.

Understanding the link between stress and female hormonal disorders is the first step toward restoring balance. It's not about eliminating stress—an unrealistic goal in our fast-paced world—but rather about managing the body's response to stress. By recognizing the signs of hormonal imbalance and taking proactive steps to mitigate stress, women can help safeguard their hormonal health and overall well-being.

In this journey toward hormonal equilibrium, it's essential to acknowledge that the body's signals are not just noise to be ignored but messages to be heeded. By tuning into these signals and responding with self-care, stress reduction techniques, and, when necessary, medical intervention, women can navigate the challenges of stress and maintain their hormonal health.

Chapter Summary

- The adrenal glands play a crucial role in the body's stress response by releasing hormones like adrenaline and cortisol.
- Adrenaline triggers the 'fight or flight' response, increasing alertness and energy. At the same time, cortisol maintains energy supply and suppresses nonessential functions during prolonged stress.
- Chronic stress can lead to sustained high cortisol levels, causing health issues due to the body's constant alertness.

- Cortisol is essential for survival, regulating metabolism and the immune response. However, its balance is vital; chronic high levels can negatively impact women's health.
- High cortisol can disrupt sleep, cause weight gain, affect mood, and influence menstrual cycles and menopause symptoms in women.
- The concept of "adrenal fatigue" is controversial, with symptoms like fatigue and sleep disturbances, but the condition lacks robust scientific evidence.
- Managing stress is vital for hormonal balance, with strategies including a healthy diet, regular exercise, mindfulness practices, adequate sleep, and social support.
- Chronic stress can disrupt female hormonal balance, affecting menstrual cycles and fertility and increasing the risk of hormonal disorders like insulin resistance and thyroid dysfunction.

7

WEIGHT, METABOLISM, AND HORMONES

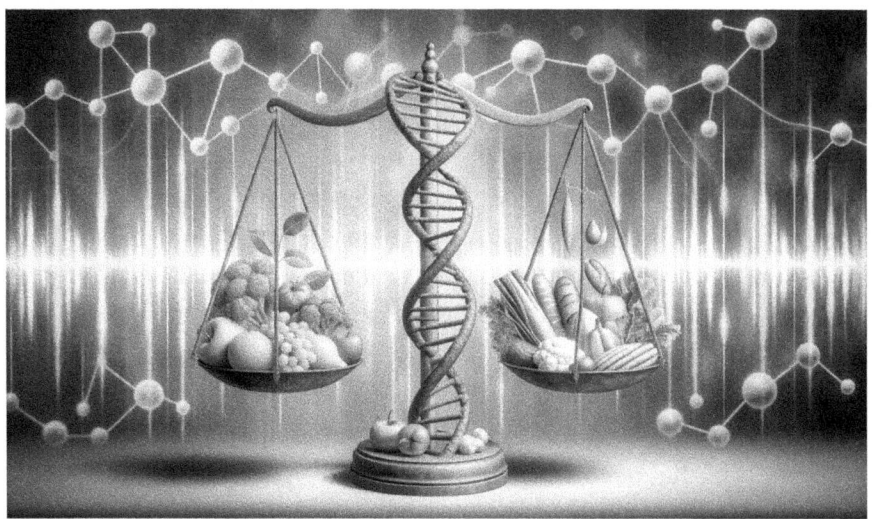

Understanding the intricate dance of hormones in your body can be like peering into a complex, ever-changing ballet. Each hormone has its role, entrance, and exit, contributing to the grand performance of your health. When it comes to weight, metabolism, and the overall energy economy of your body, hormones are the conductors, orchestrating a symphony of biological processes that can either harmonize with your health goals or, at times, seem to work against them.

One of the key players in this performance is insulin, a hormone produced by the pancreas that helps regulate blood sugar levels by facilitating glucose transport into cells for energy. Your blood sugar levels rise when you eat, signaling the pancreas to release insulin. Like a key unlocking a door, insulin allows glucose to enter the cells. As a result, your blood sugar levels begin to normalize.

However, for various reasons, sometimes the cells in your body stop responding to insulin as effectively as they should, a condition known as insulin resistance. When this happens, your pancreas works overtime, producing more insulin to get glucose into the cells. This excess insulin can have several effects on your body, including weight gain. Insulin is also known as a "storage hormone," as it signals to your body to store fat, particularly in the abdominal area, which can be especially frustrating for those trying to manage their weight.

Moreover, the relationship between insulin and weight is bidirectional. Excess body fat, particularly in the abdominal area, can increase substances known as free fatty acids, which may further promote insulin resistance. This creates a challenging cycle where weight gain can lead to more insulin resistance, which can lead to more weight gain.

But why does this happen more to some individuals than others? Genetics, lifestyle, diet, and stress levels can influence your body's sensitivity to insulin. For women, hormonal fluctuations throughout life stages, such as puberty, pregnancy, and menopause, can also impact insulin sensitivity. For instance, during menopause, the decrease in estrogen levels has been linked to an increased risk of insulin resistance.

Understanding this hormonal influence on weight is helpful because it underscores the importance of a holistic approach to weight management. It's not just about calories in versus calories out; it's about the hormonal environment within your body that affects how those calories are processed and stored.

To support healthy insulin levels and sensitivity, a balanced diet rich in fiber, healthy fats, and lean proteins can be beneficial. Regular physical activity is also key, as it can help improve insulin sensitivity by encouraging your muscles to use glucose more effectively. Additionally, managing stress and ensuring adequate sleep are important factors, as stress and sleep deprivation can negatively impact insulin sensitivity.

Remember, your body is a complex and dynamic system. While it might feel like a struggle to understand and manage the hormonal influences on your weight, know that each positive step you take is a note in the right direction, contributing to the harmony of your overall health.

Insulin Resistance and Its Impact on Health

As we delve deeper into the intricate relationship between weight, metabolism, and hormones, it's essential to understand the role of insulin resistance and its profound impact on women's health. Insulin, a hormone produced by the pancreas, is vital in managing our body's energy use. It helps cells absorb glucose from the bloodstream for energy or storage for future use. However, when insulin resistance occurs, this process becomes less efficient, and it can lead to a cascade of health issues.

Insulin resistance happens when the body's cells become less responsive to insulin. This means that despite the presence of insulin in the bloodstream, glucose remains outside the cells, leading to elevated blood sugar levels. Sensing high blood sugar, the pancreas produces even more insulin to elicit the proper cellular response. This excess insulin can create a hormonal imbalance, contributing to weight gain and difficulty losing weight.

For many women, insulin resistance is a silent condition, often going unnoticed until it manifests as prediabetes or type 2 diabetes. However, its effects on metabolism and weight can be felt long before such diagnoses. Women with insulin resistance may experience fatigue, cravings for carbohydrates, and difficulty managing their weight despite a healthy diet and exercise.

Various factors, including genetics, lifestyle choices, and hormonal changes, can influence the development of insulin resistance. Women, in particular, may face unique challenges due to hormonal fluctuations during their menstrual cycle, pregnancy, and menopause, which can all affect insulin sensitivity.

Moreover, insulin resistance is closely linked to a condition known as polycystic ovary syndrome (PCOS), which affects hormonal balance and can lead to irregular menstrual cycles, fertility issues, and weight gain. Women with PCOS often struggle with insulin resistance, which exacerbates the syndrome's symptoms and complicates its management.

Addressing insulin resistance involves a multifaceted approach. Lifestyle modifications, such as incorporating regular physical activity and adopting a balanced diet rich in fiber and low in refined sugars, can significantly improve insulin sensitivity. Sometimes, healthcare providers may recommend medication to help manage blood sugar levels.

Understanding insulin resistance is a critical step in taking control of one's hormonal health. By recognizing the signs and knowing the strategies to combat it, you can work towards restoring balance and enhancing their overall well-being. As we explore the hormonal landscape, we'll discover that hormones like leptin and ghrelin also play pivotal roles in hunger and satiety, further influencing weight and metabolism. By considering the full spectrum of hormonal interactions, we can better appreciate the complexity and interconnectedness of our body's systems.

Leptin and Ghrelin: Hunger Hormones Explained

In the intricate dance of weight management and metabolism, two key players often don't get the spotlight they deserve: leptin and ghrelin. These hormones play crucial roles in regulating hunger and satiety, acting as the body's natural messengers for when to eat and when to stop. Understanding how they work can offer us valuable insights into our relationship with food and our journey towards hormonal balance.

Leptin, often called the "satiety hormone," is produced by your fat cells. It communicates with the hypothalamus in your brain, which is the command center for appetite regulation. When you have sufficient fat stores, leptin levels increase, signaling to your brain that you have enough energy, which helps to curb your appetite. Conversely, when fat stores are low, leptin levels drop, and the brain interprets this as a sign to seek out food.

However, the story of leptin isn't always straightforward. Sometimes, despite adequate or even excessive fat stores, the brain can become less sensitive to leptin—a condition known as leptin resistance. This can lead to a perpetual feeling of hunger and overeating, as the brain doesn't receive the proper signal to stop eating. Leptin resistance is a complex issue, influenced by factors such as inflammation, high levels of fatty acids in the bloodstream, and high leptin levels itself.

On the flip side of the coin is ghrelin, the "hunger hormone," primarily produced in the stomach. Ghrelin levels rise when the stomach is empty and fall after it's filled. This hormone signals the brain that it's time to seek nourishment. If you've ever experienced those intense hunger pangs after skipping a meal, you can thank ghrelin for that urgent nudge to refuel.

The interplay between leptin and ghrelin is a delicate balance that affects not only our hunger levels but also our overall metabolic health. Disruptions in this balance can lead to weight gain and difficulty losing weight and affect energy levels and mood.

It's important to note that factors such as sleep deprivation, stress, and diet can influence the levels of these hormones. For instance, lack of sleep has been shown to decrease leptin levels and increase ghrelin, which might explain why we often feel hungrier after a poor night's sleep. Stress, too, can elevate ghrelin levels, leading to increased appetite and cravings, particularly for high-calorie comfort foods.

Understanding the roles of leptin and ghrelin can empower us to make more informed choices about our diet and lifestyle. Simple practices like getting adequate sleep, managing stress, and eating a balanced diet rich in fiber, protein, and healthy fats can help maintain the delicate balance of these hormones. Moreover, regular physical activity can improve the body's sensitivity to leptin, making it a key component in managing hunger and maintaining a healthy weight.

As we navigate the complexities of hormone health, it's clear that these hunger hormones are pivotal in the conversation about weight and metabolism. By tuning into the signals of leptin and ghrelin, we can foster a more harmonious relationship with food and support our bodies in achieving hormonal equilibrium.

The Thyroid-Weight Connection

Understanding the intricate dance between your thyroid and weight can be a revelation, especially if you've struggled with the scales despite your best efforts. The thyroid gland, a butterfly-shaped organ nestled in the front of your neck, is critical in regulating your metabolism. As we learned in earlier chapters, the thyroid produces hormones—chiefly thyroxine (T4) and triiodothyronine (T3)—that control the speed at which your body converts food into energy.

When your thyroid functions optimally, it maintains a balance that allows your metabolism to run smoothly. However, if the thyroid produces too much hormone, a condition known as hyperthyroidism, your metabolism accelerates. This can lead to weight loss, among other symptoms, but it's not a healthy or sustainable way to manage weight.

On the flip side, if your thyroid doesn't produce enough hormone—a condition called hypothyroidism—your metabolism slows down. This can lead to weight gain, and it can be frustrating because it often feels like no matter how little you eat or how much you exercise, the weight just doesn't come off.

It's essential to recognize that weight changes can be one of the first signs that your thyroid isn't functioning as it should. Women, in particular, are more susceptible to thyroid disorders, especially after pregnancy and during menopause. If you're experiencing unexpected changes in your weight, it's worth discussing with your healthcare provider whether a thyroid function test is appropriate.

Managing thyroid-related weight issues is not solely about diet and exercise; it's about getting to the root of the hormonal imbalance. If you are diagnosed with a thyroid condition, treatment typically involves hormone replacement therapy for hypothyroidism or medication to suppress hormone production for hyperthyroidism. Once your thyroid hormone levels are stabilized, your metabolism should return to a more normal rate, making managing your weight easier.

Remember, the goal is not just to reach a certain number on the scale, but to foster a healthy and balanced body. Patience is key, as it can take time for your body to adjust to new thyroid hormone levels. In the meantime, focusing on a nutrient-rich diet and regular physical activity can support overall well-being and complement any medical treatments for your thyroid.

As we move forward, we'll explore how you can proactively manage your weight by understanding and working with your body's hormonal cues. Adopting hormonal strategies for weight management can create a personalized approach that supports your body's unique needs and helps you maintain a healthy weight and metabolism.

Hormonal Strategies for Weight Management

Understanding the intricate dance of hormones and their impact on weight can be both empowering and daunting. As we've explored the significance of thyroid function in weight regulation, let's now broaden our perspective to recap some additional hormonal strategies that can aid in weight management.

Firstly, it's essential to recognize that weight management is not solely about the calories in versus calories out equation. Hormones are crucial in how your body stores fat, manages hunger and dictates energy levels. Therefore, a holistic approach to weight management should include strategies that consider hormonal balance.

One of the key players in this balance is insulin, a hormone produced by the pancreas that helps regulate blood sugar levels. When we consume foods, particularly those high in carbohydrates, our bodies break them down into glucose, which enters the bloodstream. Insulin is then released to help cells absorb and use glucose for energy. However, when insulin levels are consistently high due to a diet high in refined sugars and carbs, the body becomes less sensitive to it, a condition known as insulin resistance. This can lead to weight gain, especially around the abdomen, and increase the risk of developing type 2 diabetes.

Consider incorporating a fiber-rich diet, healthy fats, and proteins to support insulin sensitivity. These nutrients have a more gradual effect on blood sugar, which can help maintain steady insulin levels. Regular physical activity also enhances insulin sensitivity by helping the muscles absorb glucose without needing as much insulin.

Another crucial hormone for weight management is leptin, which is produced by fat cells and signals to the brain that you have enough energy stored, reducing appetite. However, just like insulin, it's possible to develop leptin resistance, where the brain no longer receives the satiety signal effectively, leading to overeating. Getting enough sleep is vital to support healthy leptin levels, as sleep deprivation can disrupt its production. Additionally, reducing inflammation through a diet rich in antioxidants from fruits, vegetables, and omega-3 fatty acids can help maintain leptin sensitivity.

Cortisol, the stress hormone, also has a significant impact on weight. Chronic stress can lead to elevated cortisol levels, which can increase appetite and drive abdominal fat storage. Managing stress through mindfulness practices, adequate sleep, and relaxation techniques can help keep cortisol levels in check.

Lastly, the balance of estrogen and progesterone can influence weight. Estrogen dominance, a condition where there is too much estrogen relative to progesterone, can lead to weight gain. To support hormonal balance, consider lifestyle changes such as reducing exposure to xenoestrogens found in plastics and certain personal care products and incorporating foods that support liver health and detoxification, like cruciferous vegetables.

In conclusion, a comprehensive approach to weight management should include dietary and exercise considerations and an understanding of how to support and balance hormones. You can create a more effective and sustainable weight management strategy that aligns with your body's natural processes by considering things like insulin sensitivity, leptin, cortisol levels, and the balance of estrogen and progesterone. Everyone's hormonal landscape is unique, so it's important to work with a healthcare provider to tailor these strategies to your needs.

Chapter Summary

- Hormones play a crucial role in weight management, metabolism, and energy regulation, with insulin being a critical hormone facilitating glucose transport into cells.
- Insulin resistance can lead to weight gain, especially abdominal fat, and is influenced by genetics, lifestyle, diet, and stress, with women experiencing additional fluctuations during life stages.
- A holistic approach to weight management should consider the hormonal environment, with a balanced diet and regular exercise improving insulin sensitivity.
- Insulin resistance is a silent condition that can lead to prediabetes or type 2 diabetes, with women facing unique challenges due to hormonal changes.
- Leptin and ghrelin are hormones that regulate hunger and satiety, with imbalances contributing to weight gain and metabolic issues.
- Sleep, stress, and diet impact leptin and ghrelin levels, affecting hunger and the ability to maintain a healthy weight.
- Thyroid hormones control metabolism, with hyperthyroidism causing weight loss and hypothyroidism leading to weight gain, particularly affecting women.
- Hormonal strategies for weight management include supporting insulin sensitivity, maintaining healthy leptin levels, managing cortisol, and balancing estrogen and progesterone.

8
MOOD, BRAIN FUNCTION, AND HORMONES

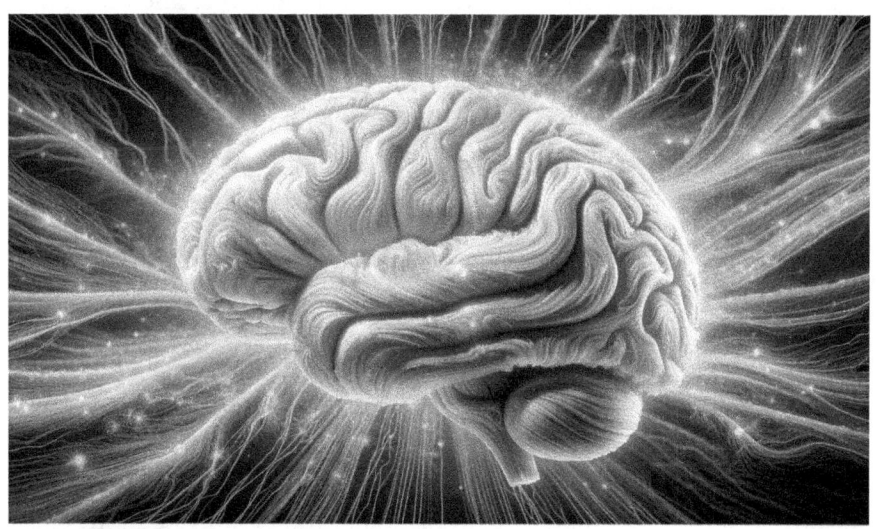

As we navigate the intricate dance of hormones within the female body, it's essential to understand their profound influence on mood. Hormones are not just chemical messengers dictating physical processes but also key players in your emotional and psychological well-being.

At the heart of this conversation is the interplay between hormones and mood. It's a complex and dynamic relationship, reflecting the ebb and flow of hormonal levels throughout life. From the onset of puberty to the transition into menopause, hormones can steer the ship of emotions, sometimes through calm waters, other times through turbulent seas.

Estrogen, one of the primary female sex hormones, has a particularly significant role in modulating mood. Fluctuations in estrogen levels can change the brain's chemistry, influencing the production and function of neurotransmitters such as serotonin, dopamine, and norepinephrine. These neurotransmitters are pivotal in regulating mood, and their balance is crucial for emotional stability.

During certain times in the menstrual cycle, particularly in the days leading up to menstruation, estrogen levels decline. Many women may experience premenstrual syndrome (PMS), which can include mood swings, irritability, and feelings of sadness. For some, these symptoms are mild and manageable. Still, for others, they can be severe and disruptive, a condition known as premenstrual dysphoric disorder (PMDD).

Pregnancy is another period of hormonal roller coaster, with estrogen and progesterone levels rising significantly. While some women feel an enhanced sense of well-being and a positive shift in mood during pregnancy, others may struggle with mood swings and even prenatal depression.

The transition to menopause, characterized by a more pronounced fluctuation and eventual decline in estrogen, can also be a time of emotional upheaval for many women. The perimenopausal period may bring about mood swings, anxiety, and depression, symptoms that can be distressing and often misunderstood.

It's not just the fluctuations that impact mood but also the brain's sensitivity to these hormonal changes. Some women may be more sensitive to shifts in estrogen and can experience more pronounced mood disturbances as a result. This sensitivity is not a sign of weakness but a reflection of the unique interplay between hormones and brain chemistry.

Understanding the hormonal underpinnings of mood is not about pathologizing the natural cycles of the female body. Instead, it's about recognizing the legitimacy of these experiences and the importance of addressing them with compassion and care. Whether through lifestyle modifications, therapeutic interventions, or medical treatments, there are many pathways to support hormone health and mood stability.

As we continue to explore the realm of female hormone health, it's clear that the mind and body are inextricably linked. The next step in our journey delves deeper into the cognitive aspects of hormonal influence, particularly how estrogen plays a role in cognitive function, memory, and overall brain health. By understanding these connections, we can better support each other in achieving physical well-being and mental and emotional harmony.

Estrogen and Cognitive Function

As we delve deeper into the intricate relationship between hormones and the female brain, it's essential to understand the role of estrogen in cognitive function. Estrogen, an essential hormone in women's health, is not only pivotal for reproductive functions but also plays a significant role in the brain's health and operation.

Estrogen's influence on cognition is multifaceted. It has been shown to have a protective effect on the brain, helping to maintain cognitive functions such as memory, attention, and problem-solving skills. This hormone interacts with neurotransmitters, the brain's chemical messengers, to enhance synaptic connectivity. It helps brain cells communicate more effectively, which is crucial for maintaining mental sharpness.

Research suggests that when estrogen levels are higher, such as the first two weeks of the menstrual cycle, some women may experience a boost in mental agility and verbal fluency. Conversely, during the latter half of the cycle, as estrogen levels decline, some may notice a slight dip in these cognitive areas. This ebb and flow is natural, but awareness can help women anticipate and understand changes in their cognitive performance throughout the month.

The impact of estrogen on the brain becomes particularly evident as women approach menopause. During this transition, the decline in estrogen can be associated with memory challenges and a decrease in the speed of cognitive processing. Some women report feelings of mental 'fogginess' during this time, which can be disconcerting. However, it's essential to recognize that this is a shared experience. Some strategies can help mitigate these effects, such as engaging in regular physical and mental exercise, maintaining a balanced diet, and, in some cases, considering hormone replacement therapy under the guidance of a healthcare professional.

Moreover, estrogen's role in brain health extends beyond cognition to mood regulation. While the previous section explored the broader impact of hormones on mood, it's worth noting that estrogen can influence the production and metabolism of neurotransmitters like serotonin and dopamine, which are directly related to mood and emotional well-being. This intricate dance between estrogen and brain chemicals is a crucial factor in understanding why some women may be more susceptible to mood swings or depression at certain times in their hormonal cycles.

Understanding estrogen's role in cognitive function is empowering. It allows you to better navigate the changes that occur throughout your life, from the menstrual cycle to menopause, and to seek support and strategies that can help maintain cognitive health and overall well-being. As we continue to explore the hormonal influences on the brain, we'll examine the connection between serotonin and premenstrual syndrome (PMS), shedding light on how hormonal fluctuations can affect emotional states in more detail.

The Serotonin Connection and PMS

As we delve into the intricate relationship between hormones and mood, it's essential to understand the role of serotonin. This critical neurotransmitter significantly influences our emotional state. For many women, the days leading up to menstruation can be marked by a cluster of physical and emotional symptoms known as premenstrual syndrome (PMS). While PMS can manifest in various ways, mood-related symptoms such as irritability, anxiety, and sadness are among the most common. They can be profoundly disruptive to a woman's daily life.

Serotonin is often called the "feel-good" neurotransmitter because it boosts mood and creates a sense of calm. It helps regulate mood, sleep, appetite, and cognition. The connection between serotonin levels and PMS symptoms is a critical piece of the puzzle when it comes to understanding how hormonal fluctuations can affect brain function and mood.

During the menstrual cycle, levels of estrogen and progesterone rise and fall. Estrogen has a modulatory effect on serotonin receptors. As such, fluctuations in estrogen levels can lead to changes in serotonin activity. In the luteal phase of the menstrual cycle, which occurs after ovulation and before menstruation begins, estrogen levels decline. This decrease can result in reduced serotonin activity, which may contribute to mood swings and other emotional symptoms associated with PMS.

Some women may be more sensitive to these hormonal changes than others, which can explain why PMS symptoms vary widely in both type and intensity. It's also worth noting that serotonin is synthesized from tryptophan, an amino acid obtained from our diet. Nutritional factors, therefore, can also play a role in serotonin levels and, by extension, PMS symptoms.

Understanding the serotonin connection to PMS offers avenues for managing the emotional symptoms. Lifestyle modifications, such as regular exercise and a balanced diet rich in tryptophan-containing foods, can help maintain stable serotonin levels. In some cases, healthcare providers may also recommend pharmacological interventions, such as selective serotonin reuptake inhibitors (SSRIs), a class of medications that can help increase serotonin activity in the brain.

It's important to approach the management of PMS with a holistic perspective, considering the biological underpinnings and the personal and emotional experiences of each individual. By acknowledging the complex interactions between hormones, brain function, and mood, we can better support women in navigating these monthly changes with greater understanding and compassion.

As we continue to explore the impact of hormones on mental health, it becomes clear that the conversation extends beyond PMS. Hormonal influences are far-reaching, potentially affecting a range of mental health disorders. By building on our knowledge of how hormones like estrogen and neurotransmitters like serotonin interact, we can deepen our understanding of mental health and work towards more effective strategies for maintaining hormonal balance and emotional well-being.

Hormones and Mental Health Disorders

In the intricate dance of hormones and mental well-being, it's essential to recognize the profound impact that hormonal fluctuations can have on mental health disorders in women. While the previous discussion highlighted the role of serotonin, a key neurotransmitter, in premenstrual syndrome (PMS), it's important to delve deeper into the broader spectrum of mental health conditions that are influenced by hormonal changes.

Hormones such as estrogen and progesterone do more than just regulate the menstrual cycle; they also play critical roles in the brain, affecting mood, cognition, and mental health. Estrogen, for example, has a protective effect on the brain and is thought to enhance mood and cognitive function. It interacts with neurotransmitters implicated in mood disorders, such as serotonin and dopamine. This is why some women may experience mood swings, depression, or anxiety in relation to their menstrual cycle, during the postpartum period, or as they transition into menopause.

Progesterone, on the other hand, has a calming effect on the brain. It is a neurosteroid that can be a natural tranquilizer, promoting sleep and relaxation. However, the sudden drop in progesterone just before menstruation or the fluctuating levels during perimenopause can contribute to mood disturbances and anxiety.

The relationship between hormones and mental health disorders becomes even more apparent when considering conditions such as premenstrual dysphoric disorder (PMDD) and perimenopausal depression. PMDD is a severe form of PMS that can significantly disrupt a woman's life, with symptoms including intense mood swings, irritability, and depression. Perimenopausal depression, on the other hand, can emerge during the menopausal transition, a time when the hormonal landscape is changing dramatically.

Moreover, thyroid hormones also play a pivotal role in mental health.

Both hyperthyroidism and hypothyroidism can manifest with symptoms that mimic mental health disorders, such as anxiety and depression. Therefore, healthcare providers must consider thyroid function when evaluating a woman presenting with mental health concerns.

It's also worth noting that hormonal contraceptives, which are widely used by women, can influence mental health. While they can stabilize hormonal fluctuations and potentially improve mood and anxiety for some, others may experience negative mood changes as a side effect. The impact of hormonal contraceptives on mental health is highly individual and emphasizes the need for personalized medical care.

Understanding the interplay between hormones and mental health is a complex yet vital part of women's health. It requires a compassionate approach that acknowledges the unique experiences of each woman. By considering the hormonal underpinnings of mental health disorders, we can pave the way for more effective, tailored treatments that address not only the psychological but also the physiological contributors to a woman's mental well-being.

As we progress, we must consider how lifestyle choices and interventions can support hormonal balance and mood regulation. Simple yet powerful lifestyle changes can often complement medical treatments, empowering women to take an active role in managing their hormonal health.

Lifestyle Choices for Hormonal Mood Regulation

In the intricate dance of hormones and emotions, knowing we are not just passive participants is empowering. Our lifestyle choices can play a pivotal role in harmonizing this delicate balance, particularly when it comes to mood regulation.

Diet, for instance, is a cornerstone of hormonal health. Foods rich in omega-3 fatty acids, such as salmon and flaxseeds, have been shown to support brain function and may help stabilize mood. Complex carbohydrates, found in whole grains and legumes, can aid in regulating blood sugar levels, which in turn can influence hormonal balance and mood. Meanwhile, limiting sugar and refined carbs is wise, which can cause spikes and dips in blood sugar and energy levels, potentially disrupting hormonal equilibrium and emotional stability.

Physical activity is another powerful tool. Regular exercise, especially aerobic activities like walking, swimming, or cycling, encourages the release of endorphins, often referred to as the body's natural mood lifters. Exercise can also help regulate the stress hormone cortisol, which, when chronically elevated, can interfere with other hormone functions.

Sleep cannot be overstated in its importance. Quality sleep is critical for the body to repair and regulate hormone production. Disrupted sleep patterns can lead to hormonal imbalances such as estrogen and progesterone, critical players in mood regulation. Establishing a calming bedtime routine and striving for 7-9 hours of sleep per night can significantly affect hormonal health.

Stress management techniques can also be beneficial, such as mindfulness meditation, yoga, or deep-breathing exercises. Chronic stress can wreak havoc on our hormonal balance, influencing cortisol levels and other hormones that affect mood. Incorporating stress-reduction practices into our daily lives can help maintain hormonal harmony and emotional well-being.

Lastly, social connections and support networks are vital. Engaging with friends, family, or support groups can provide emotional comfort and stress relief. Positive social interactions can trigger the release of oxytocin, a hormone that promotes feelings of bonding and reduces stress responses.

Integrating these lifestyle interventions can support our hormonal health and foster a more stable mood landscape. It's a proactive approach that enhances our emotional well-being and empowers us to take charge of our overall health. Remember, small, consistent changes can lead to significant improvements over time, and it's never too late to start nurturing your hormonal harmony.

Chapter Summary

- Hormones, particularly estrogen, play a significant role in women's mood regulation, influencing neurotransmitters like serotonin, dopamine, and norepinephrine.
- Fluctuations in estrogen levels can cause mood swings and conditions like premenstrual syndrome (PMS) and premenstrual dysphoric disorder (PMDD), especially before menstruation.
- Pregnancy and menopause are periods of hormonal changes that can significantly affect a woman's mood, with some experiencing mood swings, anxiety, and depression.
- Individual sensitivity to hormonal changes can lead to varying degrees of mood disturbances among women.
- Estrogen is also crucial for cognitive functions such as memory and attention, with its levels affecting mental agility and verbal fluency.
- The serotonin connection to PMS highlights the role of diet and lifestyle in managing mood-related symptoms, with options like exercise, balanced diet, and SSRIs as treatments.
- Hormonal fluctuations can impact mental health disorders beyond PMS, with estrogen and progesterone affecting mood and cognition and thyroid hormones influencing mental health.
- Lifestyle choices, including diet, exercise, sleep, stress management, and social connections, can significantly influence hormonal balance and mood regulation.

9

SKIN, HAIR, AND HORMONES

When we think of our skin, we often consider it merely as a protective barrier or an aesthetic feature. However, it's much more than that—it's a complex organ intimately connected with our internal processes, including hormones. Understanding this connection can be particularly enlightening for women, as hormonal fluctuations throughout life stages can manifest visibly on the skin.

Hormones play a significant role in the health and appearance of our skin. Estrogen and progesterone, the primary female sex hormones, influence skin thickness, wrinkle formation, and moisture. They can enhance collagen production, giving skin its youthful, supple structure. Conversely, when these hormone levels decline, such as during menopause, the skin may lose elasticity and become drier.

Testosterone, though typically considered a male hormone, is present in women as well and can have a profound impact on the skin. Excess testosterone can increase sebum production, the oily substance that can clog pores and lead to acne. This is why some women experience breakouts not just during puberty, when hormone levels fluctuate dramatically, but also at specific points in their menstrual cycle, during pregnancy, or in conditions like polycystic ovary syndrome (PCOS), where testosterone levels may be elevated.

The thyroid hormones produced by the thyroid gland also play a crucial role in skin health. They help regulate skin cell renewal. When the thyroid is overactive (hyperthyroidism) or underactive (hypothyroidism), it can lead to a variety of skin issues. Hyperthyroidism may cause warm, moist, and smooth skin, while hypothyroidism can lead to dry, rough, and cold skin.

Cortisol, the stress hormone, can also affect the skin. Chronic stress leads to prolonged cortisol elevation, which can break down collagen and elastin, the fibers that give skin firmness and elasticity. This can accelerate aging, leading to the earlier onset of wrinkles and sagging skin.

It's not just the presence of these hormones that matters, but their balance. Hormonal imbalances can lead to various skin conditions, from dryness and sensitivity to acne and hirsutism (excessive hair growth). It's a delicate dance that changes with the rhythms of life—puberty, the menstrual cycle, pregnancy, and menopause.

Understanding the skin-hormone connection is empowering. It allows women to anticipate changes in their skin and seek appropriate treatments. Lifestyle choices, such as diet, exercise, and stress management, can influence hormone levels and, by extension, skin health. Additionally, topical treatments, medications, and hormone replacement therapies can be tailored to address specific skin concerns related to hormonal changes.

Our skin reflects our inner health, including the complex symphony of hormones that play throughout a woman's life. By nurturing our hormonal health, we also care for our skin, ensuring it remains as resilient and vibrant as possible.

Acne and Hormones: Beyond the Teenage Years

As we gracefully navigate beyond the tumultuous seas of teenage years, many of us anticipate leaving particular unwelcome companions at the shore, acne being a prime candidate. Yet, for numerous women, the reality is that acne can persist or even first appear in adulthood, often leaving them perplexed and seeking answers.

Understanding the intricate dance of hormones within our bodies is crucial in unraveling the mystery of adult acne. While adolescence is notorious for hormonal upheavals, the truth is that our endocrine system continues to ebb and flow throughout our lives, influenced by factors such as the menstrual cycle, pregnancy, birth control, and the approach of menopause.

Androgens, a group of hormones that includes testosterone, often play the lead role in the story of adult acne. These hormones can cause the sebaceous glands in the skin to produce more oil, which can lead to clogged pores and the proliferation of acne-causing bacteria. For women, fluctuations in androgen levels can be particularly pronounced during certain times of the menstrual cycle, as well as in conditions such as polycystic ovary syndrome (PCOS), where androgen levels are typically higher.

But it's not just about androgens. Estrogen and progesterone also influence skin health, with estrogen known for its skin-friendly properties, such as promoting collagen production and improving skin elasticity. As these hormone levels fluctuate, so too can the clarity and overall condition of the skin.

Stress, too, can be a significant factor. It triggers the release of cortisol, a hormone that can indirectly increase androgen levels and exacerbate skin issues. This is why, during periods of high stress, you might notice a sudden flare-up of acne, even if you're well past your teenage years.

Treatment for hormonal acne in adulthood often involves a multifaceted approach. Topical treatments and good skincare habits are the first line of defense, but for many, addressing the hormonal root of the issue is vital. This may involve the use of oral contraceptives, which can help regulate hormone levels or other medications that specifically target androgens.

Lifestyle changes can also be impactful. A balanced diet, regular exercise, and stress management techniques can all help regulate hormone levels and support overall skin health. Additionally, it's important to consider the role of skincare products and routines. Non-comedogenic products that don't clog pores and gentle, non-irritating ingredients can be beneficial in managing adult acne.

Navigating the complexities of hormone health requires patience and often a touch of trial and error. It's essential to remember that each individual's hormonal landscape is unique, and what works for one person may not work for another. Consulting with healthcare professionals, such as dermatologists or endocrinologists, can provide tailored advice and treatment options.

In the journey to understand and manage adult acne, it's essential to approach the situation with kindness towards oneself. The skin is not just an external organ; it reflects the intricate internal processes that make each woman unique. By addressing hormonal health holistically, it's possible to find solutions that clear the skin and support overall well-being.

Hair Loss and Excess Hair Growth: Hormonal Influences

As we navigate the complexities of our bodies, it's clear that hormones play a pivotal role in the health and appearance of our skin and hair. For many women, hair density and distribution changes can be a source of concern and confusion. Understanding the hormonal influences behind hair loss and excess hair growth can empower us to address these issues with greater insight and compassion.

Hair loss, or alopecia, can be particularly distressing. It's not just about vanity; our hair is often tied to our identity and sense of femininity. Various hormonal factors can contribute to hair thinning in women. A common culprit is androgenetic alopecia, also known as female pattern hair loss, which is influenced by androgens, including testosterone. While androgens are typically considered male hormones, they are present in all bodies. They can affect hair follicles by shortening the growth phase of the hair cycle, leading to thinner, shorter hairs.

Another hormonal condition that can lead to hair loss is thyroid dysfunction. Both hyperthyroidism (an overactive thyroid) and hypothyroidism (an underactive thyroid) can cause hair to become thin and brittle, often resulting in diffuse hair shedding. The thyroid gland plays a crucial role in regulating metabolism and energy use in the body. When it's out of balance, hair growth can be significantly impacted.

On the flip side, some women experience hirsutism, which is the growth of coarse, dark hair in areas where men typically grow hair, such as the face, chest, and back. This condition is often linked to an excess of androgens or an increased sensitivity of hair follicles to these hormones. Polycystic ovary syndrome (PCOS) is a common hormonal disorder that can cause both hirsutism and hair thinning on the scalp due to its association with elevated androgen levels.

It's important to recognize that these hair-related changes are not just cosmetic issues but can signal underlying health concerns. They can also take a toll on emotional well-being, leading to stress and anxiety, which, in a challenging cycle, can further exacerbate hair problems. Stress hormones like cortisol can disrupt the hair growth cycle, leading to telogen effluvium, a temporary condition where hair falls out after a stressful event.

Navigating these changes requires a multifaceted approach. It often involves working with healthcare providers to diagnose and treat underlying hormonal imbalances. Additionally, lifestyle modifications, such as managing stress, can play a supportive role in improving hair health.

In the journey toward hormonal balance and hair health, it's crucial to approach the subject with kindness towards oneself. The changes you are experiencing are not a reflection of your worth or beauty. By understanding the hormonal influences on hair, you can take informed steps toward managing your hair health while nurturing your overall well-being.

Natural Approaches to Hormonal Skin and Hair Health

In the intricate dance of hormones and health, our skin and hair often reflect the inner balance—or imbalance—of our body's hormonal symphony. As we've explored the hormonal influences on hair loss and excess hair growth, it's clear that hormones play a pivotal role in our skin and hair condition. But what can we do to foster hormonal harmony naturally and, in turn, enhance the health and appearance of our skin and hair?

First and foremost, it's important to acknowledge that each individual's hormonal landscape is unique, and what works for one person may not work for another. However, several natural approaches can support overall hormone health, which may positively affect your skin and hair.

One of the simplest yet most profound changes you can make is prioritizing sleep. Quality sleep is a cornerstone of hormonal balance. During sleep, our bodies repair and regenerate, including synthesizing and regulating hormones. Aim for 7-9 hours of restful sleep per night, and consider adopting a calming bedtime routine to help signal to your body that it's time to wind down.

Stress management is another key factor. Chronic stress can wreak havoc on hormone levels, particularly cortisol, the stress hormone, which can, in turn, affect skin and hair. Techniques such as deep breathing, meditation, yoga, or a leisurely walk can help manage stress levels. They may contribute to a more balanced hormonal state.

Exercise is a powerful tool for hormonal health. Regular physical activity can help regulate insulin levels, support healthy estrogen metabolism, and boost mood-enhancing endorphins. Whether it's a brisk walk, a dance class, or weight training, find a form of exercise you enjoy and make it a consistent part of your routine.

Herbal remedies and supplements may also play a supportive role. For instance, spearmint tea has been studied for its potential to reduce androgens, like testosterone, which can contribute to hormonal acne and hirsutism. Vitex (also known as chasteberry) is another herb that's traditionally been used to support female hormonal balance. However, it's crucial to consult with a healthcare provider before starting any new supplement, especially if you have a medical condition or are taking medications.

Topical natural treatments can also be beneficial for skin and hair. For example, tea tree oil has antimicrobial properties and may help acne-prone skin when diluted and applied topically. Similarly, oils like coconut or argan oil can nourish the scalp and hair, potentially improving hair texture and strength.

Lastly, consider the role of gentle detoxification. Our bodies are equipped with natural detoxification systems, but supporting these processes through hydration, a diet rich in fiber, and detoxifying foods like cruciferous vegetables can aid in eliminating excess hormones and toxins that may be affecting your skin and hair health.

Remember, the journey to hormonal balance is often gradual, and patience is vital. Small, consistent changes can lead to significant improvements over time. By embracing these natural approaches, you're nurturing your skin and hair and supporting your overall well-being.

The Impact of Diet on Skin and Hair

In our journey through understanding the intimate relationship between our hormones and the health of our skin and hair, we've explored the natural strategies that can support this delicate balance. Now, let's delve into nutrition and its profound impact on our hormonal well-being, mainly focusing on the skin and hair.

The adage "you are what you eat" holds a kernel of truth, especially regarding our skin and hair health. The foods we consume can either support or disrupt hormonal balance, which in turn can manifest in our external appearance. A diet rich in certain nutrients can help fortify the skin and hair, making them more resilient against hormonal fluctuations.

Firstly, let's consider the role of antioxidants. These powerful substances combat oxidative stress, which hormonal imbalances can exacerbate. Foods high in antioxidants, such as berries, dark leafy greens, and nuts, can help protect the skin from the premature aging that free radicals can cause. They also support the body's natural detoxification processes, which are crucial for maintaining hormonal equilibrium.

Another key player in the diet-skin-hair connection is omega-3 fatty acids. Found in abundance in fatty fish like salmon, flaxseeds, and walnuts, omega-3s are known for their anti-inflammatory properties. Inflammation can be a response to hormonal changes, and by mitigating this response, omega-3s can help to keep skin clear and hair strong.

Protein is the building block of hair, and ensuring adequate intake is essential for hair health. Hormonal shifts can sometimes lead to hair thinning or loss, and a diet rich in high-quality protein from sources like eggs, poultry, and legumes can provide the necessary nutrients to help maintain hair strength and growth.

Furthermore, vitamins and minerals play a significant role. For instance, vitamin E in avocados and almonds can help protect the skin from damage and support its healing processes. Zinc, present in pumpkin seeds and chickpeas, is crucial for skin repair, hormone production, and regulation.

It's also important to consider the impact of certain foods and substances that might disrupt hormonal balance. High-glycemic foods, for example, can cause spikes in insulin, which may exacerbate conditions like acne. Similarly, dairy products have been linked to hormonal disturbances in some individuals. Being mindful of how these foods affect your body can guide you in making dietary choices that support your hormonal health.

Hydration, too, cannot be overstated. Water is essential for every cellular function in our bodies, including regulating hormones and maintaining skin and hair health. Ensuring adequate hydration helps to keep the skin supple and can even prevent the scalp from becoming dry and flaky.

Incorporating a balanced diet that supports hormonal health doesn't have to be a chore. It can be a delightful exploration of flavors and foods that nourish your body and bring joy and satisfaction to your meals. Remember, the journey to hormonal balance is personal, and what works for one may not work for another. It's about listening to your body, observing how it responds to different foods, and adjusting your diet.

By embracing a diet that supports hormonal balance, you're taking a proactive step towards healthier skin and hair and overall well-being. As we continue to explore the multifaceted aspects of hormone health, remember that each choice you make at the dining table can be a powerful ally in your quest for vitality and harmony within your body.

Chapter Summary

- The skin is deeply connected to hormonal processes, with hormone fluctuations like estrogen, progesterone, and testosterone affecting its health and appearance.
- Hormonal changes during life stages such as puberty, menstrual cycles, pregnancy, and menopause can visibly impact the skin, causing acne, dryness, and wrinkles.
- Testosterone can increase sebum production and lead to acne. At the same time, thyroid hormones affect skin cell renewal, with imbalances causing various skin conditions.
- Cortisol, the stress hormone, can break down skin-supporting collagen and elastin, accelerating aging and causing wrinkles and sagging skin.
- Hormonal imbalances can lead to skin conditions such as acne and hirsutism (excessive hair growth), with a balance being crucial for skin health.
- Lifestyle choices, topical treatments, medications, and hormone therapies can help manage skin concerns related to hormonal changes.
- Adult acne can persist beyond teenage years due to hormonal fluctuations, with treatment often involving a combination of skincare, medication, and lifestyle changes.
- Hair health is also influenced by hormones, with conditions like androgenetic alopecia, thyroid dysfunction affecting hair density, and hirsutism causing excess hair growth.

10
INTEGRATIVE APPROACHES TO HORMONE HEALTH

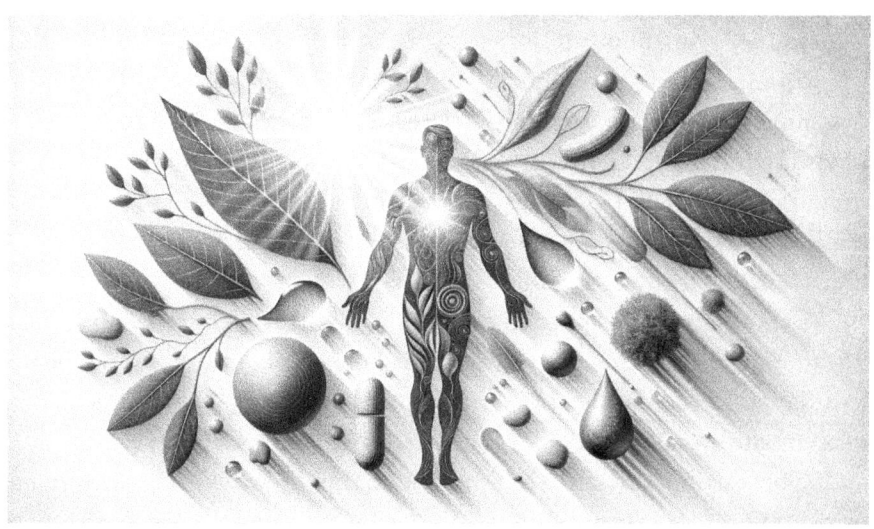

As we navigate the intricate dance of hormones within our bodies, we must recognize the profound impact our lifestyle choices have on this delicate balance.

The Role of Diet in Hormone Balance

The foods we consume can be messengers, sending signals that harmonize or disrupt our hormonal symphony.

To begin with, let's consider the building blocks of hormones: fats. Not all fats are created equal, and the quality of fats matters most. Healthy fats, such as those found in avocados, nuts, seeds, and oily fish, are necessary for hormone production and function. These fats contribute to the structural integrity of cell membranes, allowing hormones to communicate with each cell in the body effectively.

On the other hand, processed and trans fats found in many baked goods and fried foods can interfere with hormone receptors, leading to miscommunication and potential hormonal imbalances. It's like trying to have a clear conversation in a room filled with static; the message gets lost along the way.

Next, let's talk about fiber. Found in fruits, vegetables, legumes, and whole grains, fiber plays a crucial role in hormone health by aiding in the elimination of excess hormones, particularly estrogen. When estrogen levels are too high, it can lead to a variety of issues, including menstrual irregularities and mood swings. By ensuring a high-fiber diet, we support our body's natural detoxification processes, helping to maintain a harmonious hormonal environment.

Moreover, certain nutrients are pivotal in supporting hormonal health. For instance, magnesium, found in leafy greens and dark chocolate, assists in regulating cortisol, our stress hormone. B vitamins, abundant in whole grains and leafy greens, are essential for energy production and synthesizing various hormones. Vitamin D, which we can obtain from sunlight and fortified foods, is crucial for reproductive health and mood regulation.

It's also worth noting the importance of maintaining stable blood sugar levels. Frequent spikes and crashes can wreak havoc on insulin, our blood sugar-regulating hormone, and can subsequently affect other hormones such as cortisol and estrogen. To promote stable blood sugar, it's advisable to include a balanced combination of protein, healthy fats, and complex carbohydrates with each meal.

Lastly, let's not forget the role of phytoestrogens, plant-based compounds that can mimic estrogen in the body. Found in foods like soy, flaxseeds, and sesame seeds, phytoestrogens can be particularly beneficial during menopause, when the body's natural estrogen levels decline. However, the key is moderation and variety, as the effects of phytoestrogens can vary from person to person.

In summary, the foods we choose to nourish our bodies can profoundly affect our hormonal health. By focusing on whole, nutrient-dense foods and avoiding those that can disrupt hormonal communication, we lay the foundation for a balanced endocrine system. As we move forward, we'll explore how pairing these dietary choices with physical activity can enhance hormonal harmony, creating a holistic approach to health and well-being.

Exercise and Hormonal Health

In the tapestry of factors contributing to hormone health, exercise emerges as a vibrant thread, interwoven with the dietary patterns we explored earlier. Physical activity, in its many forms, profoundly impacts hormonal balance, influencing everything from stress hormones to reproductive hormones. It's a tool that, when used appropriately, can harmonize the body's endocrine symphony.

Let's begin by understanding that not all exercise is created equal in the eyes of our hormones. The type and intensity of activity can lead to different hormonal responses. For instance, moderate aerobic exercise, such as brisk walking or cycling, can boost the production of endorphins, the body's natural mood elevators. This can be particularly beneficial for women who may experience mood fluctuations associated with hormonal changes.

Resistance training, on the other hand, plays a crucial role in managing insulin sensitivity and glucose metabolism. By building lean muscle mass, women can enhance their metabolic rate, which can help regulate blood sugar levels and reduce the risk of insulin resistance—a condition that can lead to type 2 diabetes and is often associated with polycystic ovary syndrome (PCOS).

Furthermore, exercise can influence the delicate balance of estrogen and progesterone, two key players in women's reproductive health. Regular physical activity has been shown to help regulate menstrual cycles and alleviate symptoms of premenstrual syndrome (PMS) and menopause. However, it's important to note that excessive exercise or high-intensity training without adequate recovery can disrupt this balance, potentially leading to irregular periods or amenorrhea (the absence of menstruation).

Stress hormones, particularly cortisol, are also responsive to exercise. While acute bouts of exercise temporarily increase cortisol levels, chronic stress without proper rest can lead to sustained high levels of this hormone, which may disrupt overall hormonal balance. Incorporating restorative practices such as yoga or tai chi can help mitigate stress and promote a more favorable cortisol profile.

As we consider the role of exercise in hormonal health, it's essential to embrace a personalized approach. Each woman's body is unique, and what constitutes a harmonizing activity for one may not have the same effect for another. Listening to one's body and responding to its cues is paramount. This means adjusting exercise routines to align with energy levels, menstrual cycles, and life's demands.

In this journey towards hormonal equilibrium, it's also important to remember that rest is as vital as activity. Just as we need sleep to restore and rejuvenate (a topic we'll delve into more deeply in the following section), our bodies require downtime to repair and adapt to the beneficial stresses imposed by exercise.

In summary, integrating exercise into our lives is not just about pursuing fitness; it's about nurturing our hormonal health. By choosing activities that resonate with our bodies and lifestyles and balancing exertion with rest, we can use exercise as a powerful ally in achieving hormonal harmony.

Sleep's Influence on Hormonal Regulation

As we nestle into the comforting embrace of a good night's sleep, our bodies embark on an intricate dance of hormonal regulation and rebalancing. This nightly ritual is not merely about rest and recovery; it's a critical time for our endocrine system to perform essential maintenance that impacts our overall hormone health.

The relationship between sleep and hormones is a reciprocal one. Just as our hormone levels can influence how well we sleep, the quality and quantity of our sleep can profoundly affect our hormonal balance. This balance is particularly delicate and significant for women, as it governs everything from menstrual cycles to mood regulation.

One of the most well-known sleep-related hormones is melatonin, often called the "sleep hormone." Produced by the pineal gland in the brain, melatonin helps regulate our sleep-wake cycle, signaling to our bodies when it's time to wind down and prepare for sleep. Exposure to light at night can suppress melatonin production, which is why it's recommended to reduce screen time before bed to encourage a healthy sleep cycle.

But melatonin is just the beginning. Sleep also influences other hormones that are pivotal in women's health. For instance, during sleep, the body can regulate cortisol. High cortisol levels can disrupt various bodily functions, including menstrual regularity and ovulation. Women can help keep cortisol levels in check by ensuring adequate sleep and promoting a sense of calm and stability throughout the body.

Growth hormone is another key player during sleep. It helps repair and regenerate cells, supports muscle growth, and aids in the metabolism of fats. This hormone is primarily secreted during deep sleep, highlighting the importance of the duration and quality of sleep we get each night.

Furthermore, sleep impacts insulin, the hormone responsible for regulating blood sugar levels. Poor sleep can lead to insulin resistance, which can increase the risk of diabetes and weight gain. For women, particularly those with polycystic ovary syndrome (PCOS), managing insulin levels through adequate sleep is crucial for maintaining hormonal equilibrium.

Leptin and ghrelin, the hormones associated with hunger and satiety, are also influenced by our sleep patterns. A lack of sleep can lead to an increase in ghrelin, the hunger hormone, and a decrease in leptin, which signals fullness. This imbalance can result in increased cravings and a tendency to overeat, making sleep a vital component of weight management and metabolic health.

For women navigating the ebb and flow of hormonal changes throughout their lives, from menstruation to menopause, sleep becomes an essential foundation for hormonal health. It's a time for the body to reset, rebalance, and restore itself.

Establishing a consistent sleep routine is vital to harnessing the power of sleep for hormonal regulation. This includes going to bed and waking up at the same time each day, creating a restful sleep environment, and engaging in relaxing activities before bedtime. Women can support their hormonal health and enhance their overall well-being by prioritizing sleep.

As we continue exploring integrative approaches to hormone health, it becomes clear that the mind and body are interconnected. The practices that support our mental and emotional states can profoundly affect our hormonal balance. With this understanding, we can appreciate the holistic nature of our health and the various ways we can nurture it.

Mind-Body Practices for Hormonal Harmony

As we journey through the landscape of hormone health, we must recognize the profound connection between our minds and bodies. This connection is not just poetic—it's physiological. The symphony of hormones that influences everything from our mood to our metabolism is highly sensitive to our mental and emotional states. Embracing mind-body practices can be a powerful way to promote hormonal harmony.

One of the most accessible and effective mind-body practices is meditation. Meditation has been shown to reduce stress, which can help regulate cortisol levels. Cortisol can wreak havoc on other hormones when it's chronically elevated. By incorporating a daily meditation practice, even if it's just for a few minutes, you can create a space of calm within your day. This tranquility signals to your endocrine system that all is well, allowing your body to maintain a more balanced hormonal state.

Yoga, another integrative practice, combines physical postures, breath control, and meditation. It's particularly beneficial for women's hormone health because it reduces stress and supports the endocrine system through specific poses that can stimulate or soothe various glands. For instance, poses like forward folds can calm the adrenal glands, while shoulder stands may invigorate the thyroid. Yoga's holistic approach nurtures the entire body and mind, fostering an environment where hormones can flourish in balance.

Deep breathing exercises, or pranayama in the yogic tradition, are also invaluable. Deep, diaphragmatic breathing activates the parasympathetic nervous system, responsible for the 'rest and digest' state. This state is crucial for allowing the body to repair and regulate itself, including hormonal functions. By practicing deep breathing, you can help reduce the fight-or-flight response triggered by stress and encourage a more harmonious hormonal milieu.

Biofeedback is a more technologically advanced mind-body technique that can also aid in managing hormone health. It involves using electronic monitoring to convey information about physiological processes. With this feedback, you can learn to control certain bodily functions that are usually involuntary, like heart rate or muscle tension. Over time, biofeedback can teach you to mitigate your body's stress response and improve conditions like PMS or menopausal symptoms, which are often exacerbated by stress.

Lastly, mindfulness can be woven throughout your day to maintain a state of hormonal equilibrium. Mindfulness involves being fully present and engaged in the moment without judgment. This can mean savoring your food, which can help with digestive hormones, or being fully attentive during conversations, reducing stress and improving your emotional well-being.

Incorporating these mind-body practices into your life doesn't require a complete lifestyle overhaul. It's about finding moments to pause, breathe, and connect with yourself throughout your day. By doing so, you're not just nurturing your mind but taking an active role in your hormone health. As we move forward, remember that the journey to hormonal health is about what we put into our bodies and how we tune into our internal rhythms and cultivate inner peace.

Navigating Hormone Therapy and Supplements

As we delve into the realm of hormone therapy and supplements, it's essential to approach this topic with a blend of caution, curiosity, and a deep respect for the intricate symphony of your body's hormonal system. Hormone therapy and the use of supplements can be powerful tools in the quest for hormonal balance. Still, they have their complexities and potential risks.

When considering hormone therapy, it's essential to understand that this approach often involves replacing or supplementing hormones in your body to alleviate symptoms associated with hormonal imbalances or deficiencies. This can be particularly relevant during life transitions such as perimenopause and menopause or in conditions like hypothyroidism or polycystic ovary syndrome (PCOS).

However, hormone therapy is not a one-size-fits-all solution. It requires a personalized approach, often starting with comprehensive testing to determine your specific hormonal needs. Blood, saliva, or urine tests can provide a snapshot of your hormonal landscape, guiding your healthcare provider in tailoring a treatment plan for you.

When it comes to hormone replacement therapy (HRT), there are several options available, including bioidentical hormones, which are chemically identical to those your body produces naturally. These can come in various forms, such as pills, patches, creams, or gels. The decision to use bioidentical hormones should be made in collaboration with a healthcare professional who can help weigh the benefits against potential risks, such as the increased risk of certain cancers or cardiovascular events associated with some forms of HRT.

Supplements, on the other hand, can offer a more indirect approach to supporting hormone health. They can include a range of vitamins, minerals, herbs, and other nutraceuticals that may help to support the body's natural hormone production and balance. For instance, vitamin D and magnesium are crucial for bone health, especially as estrogen levels decline during menopause. Omega-3 fatty acids can support mood and reduce inflammation. At the same time, adaptogenic herbs like ashwagandha may help the body cope with stress and support adrenal health.

It's vital to approach supplements with the same level of scrutiny as any other treatment. Not all supplements are created equal, and their quality can vary widely. It's advisable to look for products that have been third-party tested for purity and potency. Furthermore, discussing any supplements you're considering with your healthcare provider is essential, as they can interact with medications and may not be appropriate for everyone.

Remember, hormone therapy and supplements are just one piece of the puzzle. They can be effective when used judiciously and in conjunction with other lifestyle interventions, such as a balanced diet, regular exercise, adequate sleep, and stress management techniques. Your body is a complex and dynamic system, and nurturing hormone health is a journey that often requires a multifaceted approach.

As you navigate the options available to you, keep in mind that your journey is unique. What works for one person may not work for another. It's about finding harmony within your body and working with healthcare professionals who listen to you, understand your goals, and help you make informed decisions about your hormone health. With patience and persistence, you can find a path that addresses your symptoms and enhances your overall well-being.

Chapter Summary

- Dietary choices significantly influence hormonal balance, with certain foods acting as messengers that can harmonize or disrupt the endocrine system.
- Healthy fats are essential for hormone production and function, while processed and trans fats can interfere with hormone receptors.
- Fiber aids in eliminating excess hormones, particularly estrogen, and supports the body's natural detoxification processes.

- Nutrients like magnesium, B vitamins, and Vitamin D are pivotal for regulating stress hormones, energy production, and reproductive health.
- Maintaining stable blood sugar levels is crucial for hormonal balance, and a diet balanced with protein, fats, and complex carbs can help.
- Phytoestrogens found in foods like soy and flaxseeds can mimic estrogen in the body and are beneficial in moderation, especially during menopause.
- Exercise impacts hormonal health, with different types and intensities of activity influencing stress and reproductive hormones.
- Adequate sleep is critical for hormonal regulation, affecting hormones like melatonin, cortisol, growth hormone, insulin, leptin, and ghrelin.

YOUR HORMONAL JOURNEY

As we conclude this book, it's time to reflect on our journey together. We've navigated the complex landscape of the endocrine system, uncovering how hormones influence every aspect of a woman's health. From the onset of puberty to the transition to menopause, we've explored the pivotal moments that define the hormonal experience of womanhood.

This journey has revealed the delicate balance hormones bring to our lives, impacting our physical well-being, emotional states, and mental clarity. We've learned that small messengers can have powerful effects and that understanding their language is vital to maintaining our health. The knowledge gained here serves as a foundation for building a more attuned relationship with your body.

We've also seen that hormonal imbalances are not destinies set in stone but are challenges that can be met with informed strategies and compassionate self-care. Recognizing the signs of imbalance and responding with appropriate interventions can steer your health toward equilibrium.

The journey continues after the last page of this book. It's an ongoing process of listening to your body, adapting to its needs, and advocating for your well-being. As you continue to grow and change, so will your hormonal needs. With the insights and tools you've acquired, you're better prepared to face those changes confidently and gracefully. Remember, your hormonal health is a personal voyage that you navigate with the wisdom and understanding you've gathered along the way.

Celebrating Empowerment and Self-Care

The voyage through this book has been one of discovery and empowerment. By delving into the intricacies of the endocrine system and its profound impact on every facet of your life, you've taken an important step towards self-care and personal well-being. This book has aimed to arm you with the knowledge to become an advocate for your health, understanding that hormonal balance is a cornerstone of your overall vitality.

Empowerment comes from recognizing that you have the tools and information to influence your hormonal health positively. You've learned about the importance of diet, exercise, stress management, and sleep—each a powerful lever in your control. By making conscious choices in these areas, you can support your endocrine system and enhance your quality of life.

Self-care is an act of self-love, and by prioritizing it, you honor your body's needs. The practices and insights shared in this book encourage you to listen to your body's signals and respond with nurturing actions. Whether through a nourishing meal, a rejuvenating workout, or a moment of mindfulness, each act of self-care is a celebration of your commitment to your health.

As you continue on your path, remember that self-care is not a destination but a journey that requires patience, kindness, and perseverance. Celebrate each step you take and each choice you make in favor of your well-being. The empowerment you've gained through this journey is a testament to your strength and dedication to living a balanced and healthy life.

The Future of Your Hormonal Health

As you close the final chapter, it's essential to look forward to the future of your hormonal health with optimism and a proactive mindset. The journey to understanding and managing your hormones is an evolving process that will continue to unfold as you move through life's stages and face new challenges.

The field of hormone health is dynamic, with ongoing research and advancements that promise to deepen our understanding and improve our approaches to care. Staying abreast of these developments is crucial, as they may offer new insights into treatments, therapies, and preventative measures that can further enhance your well-being.

Your hormonal health journey is also subject to change. Your hormonal needs will evolve as your body ages and your life circumstances shift. This book has equipped you with a solid foundation, but it's essential to remain vigilant and responsive to your body's cues. Regular check-ups with healthcare professionals, staying informed about your options, and making lifestyle adjustments as necessary are all part of maintaining hormonal balance over time.

Embrace the future with the knowledge that you are not a passive participant in your hormonal health. You have the power to influence it through the choices you make every day. Whether through nutrition, exercise, stress management, or medical intervention, you have the tools to support your endocrine system and thrive. The future of your hormonal health is bright, and with the wisdom you've gained, you're well-prepared to meet it head-on.

Continue Learning and Growing

The conclusion of this book is not an end but a call to action—a beckoning towards continued learning and growth in your hormonal health journey. The empowerment you've gained through understanding your hormones and endocrine system is just the beginning. It's a foundation upon which you can build a lifetime of well-being, adapting to the ever-changing landscape of your body's needs.

I urge you to remain curious and proactive. Seek out new information, stay updated with the latest research, and consider how emerging science can benefit your personal health narrative. Your body is a living library of signals and symptoms; learning to read and interpret these cues is a skill that will serve you well throughout your life.

Engage with communities that share your commitment to hormonal health. Whether through online forums, local support groups, or wellness workshops, connecting with others provides a wealth of shared knowledge and mutual encouragement. These networks can be invaluable resources as you navigate the complexities of hormonal balance.

Remember, your journey is unique; what works for one may not work for another. Be willing to experiment, to listen to your body, and to adjust your approach as necessary. Your path to hormonal harmony is one of personal evolution, requiring patience, resilience, and an open mind.

Take this call to action to heart. Continue to learn, to grow, and to thrive. Your health is a lifelong quest, and with each step, you grow stronger and more attuned to your body's needs. Embrace this journey with confidence and the knowledge that you can cultivate the vibrant health you deserve.

Nurturing Your Hormonal Balance Beyond the Pages

As we part ways, I extend to you heartfelt words of support and encouragement. This book has been a vessel of knowledge, a guide through the sometimes turbulent waters of hormonal health, but the journey doesn't end here. It continues with each day you commit to understanding and nurturing your body.

Remember, you are not alone on this path. Countless women are on similar journeys, each with a story of challenges and triumphs. Draw strength from this collective experience and know your efforts to achieve hormonal balance are important and shared.

Take pride in the steps you've already taken. Whether minor adjustments or significant changes, each one is a victory in its own right. Celebrate your progress and be gentle with yourself when faced with setbacks. Hormonal health is not about perfection; it's about striving for balance and well-being within the beautiful complexity of your body.

I encourage you to hold onto the hope and determination that have brought you this far. Continue to advocate for your health with the wisdom and tools you've acquired. Your journey is one of empowerment, a testament to your resilience and dedication to living your best life.

As you move forward, carry with you the knowledge that you are capable, strong, and fully equipped to navigate the ever-changing landscape of your hormonal health. May this book remain a trusted friend, and you step into the future with confidence and grace. Your path to hormonal harmony is yours to shape, and I am cheering for you at every step.

EPILOGUE

As we close the final pages of "Harmonize and Thrive," a collection that weaves together "Sync Your Cycle" and "Woman's Hormone Handbook," I hope that you stand at the threshold of a new beginning. This is not the end of a journey but rather the commencement of a profound relationship with your body, a continuous dialogue between your inner world and the life you lead.

Throughout "Sync Your Cycle," we explored the delicate dance of your menstrual cycle, a rhythm as natural and significant as the changing tides. You've learned to chart the ebb and flow of your hormones, to recognize the subtle cues that each phase presents, and to align your lifestyle with these biological rhythms. The knowledge you've gained is a testament to the power of living in sync with your cycle, a celebration of the strength and resilience that comes from understanding your body's innate wisdom.

In "Woman's Hormone Handbook," we delved into the intricate tapestry of hormonal health, unraveling the threads that weave together the story of womanhood. From the first whispers of puberty to the transformative waves of menopause, you've been equipped with the tools to navigate the complexities of your endocrine system. This book has illuminated the path to hormonal harmony, empowering you to take control of your well-being and embrace each stage of life with confidence and grace.

As you step forward, remember that the knowledge contained within these pages is more than just information—it is a catalyst for transformation. The practices and insights you've discovered are designed to be integrated into your daily life to become as natural and habitual as breathing. Your body is a living, breathing ecosystem, and you are its compassionate caretaker, attuned to its needs and rhythms.

The end of "Harmonize and Thrive" is an invitation to continue nurturing the seeds of wisdom you've planted. It is an encouragement to remain curious, to keep learning and growing, and to extend the compassion you've cultivated for yourself to others who may benefit from your journey. Share your experiences, challenges, and victories, for in doing so, you contribute to a collective understanding and a community of support.

Remember, the path to harmony is not linear, nor is it without its obstacles. There will be days when you feel out of sync, when the knowledge you've gained seems to slip through your fingers. In those moments, be gentle with yourself. Return to the principles you've learned, reach out for support, and trust in the resilience of your body. Your cycle is a spiral, a journey that circles back on itself, offering endless opportunities for growth and renewal.

My greatest wish is for "Harmonize and Thrive" to be a trusted companion on your path to wellness. Let it be a source of comfort and inspiration, a reminder that you are not alone in your quest for balance and vitality. Your story is a part of a larger narrative, one that encompasses the experiences of women across the globe and throughout history.

In the end, "Harmonize and Thrive" is more than a collection of books —it is a movement, a chorus of voices rising together to celebrate the power and potential of the female body. As you move forward, carry with you the knowledge that you are part of this chorus, a vital note in the symphony of womanhood.

Harmonize and Thrive

Thank you for embarking on this journey with me. May you continue to harmonize and thrive today, tomorrow, and in all the adventures to come.

Your Feedback Matters

As we reach the end of this book, I extend my heartfelt gratitude for your time and engagement. It's been an honor to share this journey with you, and I hope it has been as enriching for you as it has been for me.

Your feedback benefits me as an author and guides fellow readers in their quest for their next meaningful read. Your insights and reflections are invaluable; by sharing them, you contribute to a larger conversation that extends far beyond the pages of this book.

If the ideas we've explored have sparked new thoughts, inspired change, or provided comfort, I'd really appreciate it if you could share your experience with others by leaving a review on the platform you purchased this book from. Alternatively, you can follow the QR code below.

Thank you once again for your company on this literary adventure. May the insights you've gained stay with you, and may your continuous quest for knowledge be ever-fulfilling.

ABOUT THE AUTHOR

Lila Lacy is a passionate advocate for women's health and well-being. With years of experience working in women's health advocacy, Lila has dedicated her career to empowering women through knowledge and support.

Her journey began with a deep interest in the intricate dance of hormones within the female body and how they influence every aspect of health and daily life. Recognizing the lack of accessible, comprehensive information on the subject, Lila set out to bridge the gap between medical research and the everyday experiences of women.

Lila writes with the conviction that understanding one's body is the first step toward wellness and self-empowerment. Her work is characterized by its empathetic tone, practical advice, and unwavering commitment to debunking myths surrounding women's health.

Lila Lacy continues to be a beacon of hope and a source of cutting-edge information for women seeking to reclaim their health and harmony with their bodies. Her books not only educate but also inspire readers to make lasting changes that resonate through all facets of their lives.

When she's not writing or speaking, Lila enjoys practicing yoga, experimenting with hormone-friendly recipes, and spending time in nature.

www.ingramcontent.com/pod-product-compliance
Lightning Source LLC
Chambersburg PA
CBHW051539020426
42333CB00016B/1999